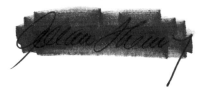

The Poetry
of Healing

THE
POETRY
OF
HEALING

*A Doctor's Education
in Empathy, Identity,
and Desire*

RAFAEL CAMPO

W. W. NORTON & COMPANY
New York   London

The text of this book is composed in Weiss Roman
with the display set in Weiss Titling and Weiss Italic.
Desktop composition by Gina Webster using QuarkXpress 3.31
Manufacturing by The Haddon Craftsmen, Inc.
Book design by Charlotte Staub

Library of Congress Cataloging-in-Publication Data
Campo, Rafael.
The poetry of healing : a doctor's education in empathy, identity, and
desire / Rafael Campo.
    p.   cm.
ISBN 0-393-04009-7
1. Campo, Rafael. 2. Hispanic American physicians—United
States—Biography. 3. Poets—United States—Biography.
4. Gay men—United States—Biography. I. Title.
R154.C26A3   1997
610'.92—dc20
[B]   96-23121
                                                              CIP

W. W. Norton & Company, Inc., 500 Fifth Avenue, New York, N.Y. 10110
http://www.wwnorton.com

W. W. Norton & Company Ltd., 10 Coptic Street, London WC1A 1PU
1   2   3   4   5   6   7   8   9   0

for Marilyn and Eve, who live

for Gary, who died

for Alane, who long believed

for my parents, and Jorge,

who made possible what I did ⟶

Acknowledgments

Some of these essays have appeared
previously, in slightly different form, in the
Boston Review, DoubleTake, the *Kenyon Review,*
the *New York Times Magazine,* and *Ploughshares.*
R.C.

Contents ~

The Poetry
of Healing

The Desire
to Heal ~

His erection startled me. At first, it seemed merely to point me out, acknowledging my part in the simple and various human desires present in our encounter: the desire to be loved and to be healed, the desire to be naked before another and thus to be utterly understood and to be wordlessly explained, the desire for a life beyond this one, the desire to represent what is the truth. What could be more natural than that I was there, a witness to another man's ailing body. For a fleeting moment, I too wished to be naked, to be as available to him in his suffering as he had made himself to me. The sheer exclamation of the pleasure in one person's touching the body of another—I have been a doctor long enough to know what joy and power there is in the laying on of hands—must have frightened me, so explicit and insistent it was in this form. Gradually, I let myself become aware of my stethoscope, my white coat, my cold hands in their latex gloves as they all continuously emitted their signals. The entire milieu of my chilly, fluorescently lit office seemed to be warning us both of my very great distance. I watched as if from behind a surveillance camera of my years of medical training as I mutated into an alien space scientist, studying and cataloging a curious life-form on a forbidding planet. Then I excused myself abruptly, saying in an oddly flat voice that I needed to get more liquid nitrogen to finish burning off the warts. I let the door slam shut loudly, definitively, behind me.

In considering later what had occurred between this patient of mine and me, I found myself revisiting what had drawn me to medicine in the first place. Before I was completely aware of it, I had begun to write feverishly at my cluttered desk, allowing myself to feel the presence of his body again, to touch his fragrant skin—I suddenly recalled his spicy cologne—without the barrier of my rubbery gloves. Whether it was another poem, or a long love letter, or the beginning of this book, I cannot be sure. What I do know is that in the act of writing I encountered again the shocking, empowering energy of a great desire. A desire that I have always known belongs to all of us.

My earliest conscious recollections of disturbances within my own body are those of the minor bumps and bruises whose pain was alleviated by my parents' kisses. Kissing was the most potent and intoxicating of all elixirs. Pure physical contact had the power to cure. My body, before I was capable of truly hurting myself, could be reconstituted with my mother's moist breath in my ear as she sang me a comforting song. The pleasures I felt, more intelligible to the child's mind than my parents likely suspected, are in great part what led me later in life to the healing arts. I desired to be made well in their eyes, to be acceptable, to be beautiful, to be kissed. My desiring of my parents had a good deal of its expression in the ritual of the tearfully extended, oftentimes exaggerated "boo-boo," presented for their fastidious attention. To be well meant to be well loved.

Music and magic, and particularly their expression and absorption in the physical body, were the primary modes of healing recoverable in the bits and shreds of Cuban culture that I encountered as a child. My grandmother's dark bedroom, its windows covered by thick red velvet draperies as if to keep out the weak winter light and the images of scrawny trees, seemed a shrine dedicated to the various saints before whom she lit candles as offerings. I would hear her praying or singing quietly in Spanish, believing perhaps that she was restoring health to an infirm relative back in Cuba whom she would never see again. Though I could not understand most of what she said, I let my heart be carried by her evident hope that her words could reach across the oceans. In her songs, my mind was transported all the way from sickly Elizabeth,

New Jersey, and its bleak refineries and landfills, to the verdant, lush Cuban countryside I imagined was her real home. Healing had a voice, and seemed rooted in a most potent physical longing, a longing to be with the ones you loved. Later in childhood, my family's Venezuelan maid Bonifacia would make special potions from tropical juices and other secret ingredients for me and my brothers. Some potions caused laughter; others could restore friendship or ease the pain of a lost pet. I still believe in the inherent magical properties of her concoctions, just as I understand the placebo effect: she too taught me that healing is a consequence in some measure of what the mind desires.

As I grew older, the connections multiplied between doctoring and desire. At around the age of eight, my cousins, friends, and I began "playing doctor." This enactment of adulthood was all the permission we needed to examine our own and each other's genitals freely and without shame. Though the myriad implications of our sexual acts were not yet within the realms of our conscious imaginations, we did guess capably at what might fit where. Fingers to vagina, penis to anus, mouth to nipple, each combination we employed shedding more light on the body's functions and sources of pleasure. Listening to the heart, ear pressed to the bare chest of a playmate, was the opening of a vast interior world. What did another person contain? The ingredients listed in our nursery rhymes— sugar, snails, spice, and puppy dog tails—seemed unlikely, even impossible. Whatever really constituted a person, the essence of the body felt very, very good.

At around the same time, I began to learn to fear what another's heart might contain. I recall the particular experience of playing doctor with my best friend, and his mother discovering us with our pants down in a hall closet, flashlights pointed at each other's dicks. She screamed, and angrily beat my friend before my eyes with one of the flashlights—the very instrument of our mutual and brief enlightenment. Our happy curiosity and arousal were suddenly transformed and redefined as shameful in a moment's judgment. Our queerness was apparent, revolting, and indisputable. The bandages in which we wrapped my friend afterward were blindingly white, the blood stains that soaked through them were grotesquely real, the iodine made him wince and cry visible tears. The body now bore the imprint of pain, bruises and welts written upon the skin like a language all too terribly familiar. Healing also had its origins in injury and insult, and so was a potentially painful process, not a uniformly pleasurable one. Desire had its consequences.

Just as the body could be made legible by violence, I also came to learn that the body itself could write upon the world. It could remake its very form. My own body changed under the influence of puberty's hormonal surge and lifting weights. On the soccer field, my movements became more purposeful and effective, and my approach to the sport took on the quality of narrative, as if through a game a story could be told, a deeper meaning expressed. Hair and muscle sprang up on me, announcing my sex ever more urgently. I walked differently, advertising myself to other teenagers. My penis enlarged, and demanded much more of my attention. I grasped it like a megaphone, ready to shout at the top of my lungs as I came how unimaginably wonderful it felt. A few of my friends and I masturbated together, boastfully comparing the sizes of our dicks but never daring to touch one another.

It is not surprising, then, that it was during adolescence, as my body began to speak more boldly its language of desire to the outside world, that I also began to understand medicine as a "desirable" profession. My parents, dedicated as they were to ensuring their children's security and success, urged me to consider a career as a physician. As a child of immigrants, I imagined that my white coat might make up for, possibly even purify, my nonwhite skin; learning the medical jargon might be the ultimate refutation of any questions about what my first language had been. Meanwhile, medicine was becoming a force in shaping (or in cleaning up) the culture, through government-sponsored public health messages about smoking, exercise, and drugs that filtered into my consciousness. Dr. Ruth became wildly popular, her strong German accent communicating her scientific detachment and clinical coolness. Gym and sex education classes took on a distinctly wholesome tone, intent on sanitizing our minds and bodies. Stodgy gray-haired physicians who practiced in our upper-middle-class community came to school and gave solemn talks to assemblies in the gleaming multipurpose room about VD and the evils of smoking pot.

I memorized biology homework assignments full of meiosis, gametocytes, zygotes, and stark reproduction: perhaps science could pin down the definition of desire, I thought with a mixture of hope and terror. In Sunday school lessons I had learned about Adam and Eve, and read Genesis; the biblical Eden in which they dwelled was unfailingly depicted as brightly hygienic, obsessively neat, and monotonously sunny. Their secular counterparts were laden with an equally insidious morality, the suburban white couples with emerald green lawns who were my family's neighbors, who shared our near-paradise of flowering trees that bore inedible fruit and sparkling undrinkable chlorinated pools. In science class, alongside their children I dissected frogs and cats beneath the sterile fluorescent lights, and all our instruments were autoclaved at the end of the day. I remember laying open the reproductive organs; how tidy, glistening and clean the pickled genitals seemed. The body, I was taught, was the most immaculate of machines.

When a beautiful young woman in my class with long red hair got body lice, a sort of panic ensued in our high school. It was as though a witch had been discovered, and when her parents burned her favorite jeans and black concert T-shirts, and then had her head shaved, our teachers appeared to be relieved and pleased. The message of this group hysteria seemed to be that the purpose of the body was healthful reproduction, and a relentless self-control over its processes and smallest environments was the only business of life. The pathologizing of not only tobacco and alcohol but also out-of-control, "dirty," and "addictive" consumption of sexual pleasure and food became the other side of the medical coin.

By my junior year my favorite teacher in high school was Mr. H., a middle-aged man with graying temples and an evident passion for his subject matter. He taught Advanced Placement Biology and was building an electron microscope himself. He was not exactly handsome; I recall other teachers commenting once that he was "smarmy." His hands and his veined arms would become covered in chalk dust as he diagrammed anatomical structures. After school, he dirtied himself with black grease assembling his microscope. When he taught us, he engaged us with his entire formidable body, running frantically up and down the aisles, heaving his chest as he bellowed out questions, coaxing answers out from even the shyest of mouths. His lectures were more invigorating and draining than the calisthenics of gym class. Surely no one failed to notice his tremendous bulging crotch, his tight polyester pants stretched almost painfully over his obvious hard-on. He injected a sexual energy into the classroom to which I was unaccustomed and attracted. We learned insatiably from him. He transfused the lifeblood of his risky enthusiasm into our anemic textbooks.

Mr. H. never was the hygienic physician clad in a spotless white coat that Marcus Welby was portrayed to be. His poorly concealed affair with a female classmate of mine was eventually made public by them both, to the young woman's parents and to Mr. H.'s wife (from whom we all later learned he had been long separated). Mr. H.

was asked to resign the next day, despite strident protests from the students in his classes. The humiliation and dejection in his eyes was apparent as he made his chaste announcement. Science became an ever more frightening arena indeed, where matters of the heart, excepting of course its laborious physiology, were disallowed entirely and, if pursued, led to the sternest of punishments. Passion could and indeed must be regulated, and especially the excited intercourse between teacher and student, scientist and layperson, and by extension, I began to suspect, between the mythic physician and his vulnerable patient.

In this environment I too became enraged and indignant upon reading the increasingly frequent and prurient reports in the media of chemistry teachers molesting their impressionable students, psychiatrists seducing their hypnotized subjects, and dentists fondling their anesthetized patients. A facile self-righteousness arose in me, paralleling my growing awareness of my differentness from those around me. I began imagining myself as the model physician, for whom desire was forbidden and in fact repellent, which served to defend me from my growing and undeniable sexual interest in other men. I thought I could cure myself of my own emerging identities; perhaps drinking too much guava nectar and listening too intently to merengues had made me too obviously Cuban, or masturbating too much had made me gay. I had nearly come full circle in my beliefs. In my fear of what I might become, and in accordance with what I had been taught, I reinterpreted the body as

designed for orderly reproduction and not love or pleasure, for harboring low levels of cholesterol and triglyc-
erides, not the rich voice of the soul. My grandmother,
my parents, Bonifacia, and my queer playmates disinte-
grated in the bright glare of my self-examination.

I lost twenty pounds as a premed during my sophomore
year of college; the more I desired anything, especially the
man who has since become my lover of the past eleven
years, the less I permitted myself to eat. At the same time,
I exercised obsessively, so that I was utterly exhausted at
the end of each day. Though I studied my premedical
course materials frantically, I loathed the thought of visiting a doctor for the worsening pain in my left upper
abdomen. After a prolonged period of time around
midterms when my increasing intake of Diet Coke and
Marlboros precluded that of food—my base appetites
were almost completely suppressed—I felt a pain in my
left side so sharp I forced myself to dial Campus
Emergency. Minutes later, lying naked except for a flimsy
gown on one of the Student Health Services examining
room tables, I had a fantasy that was almost overpowering
in its vividness. My attending physician was an older Mr.
H., and though his strong physical presence seemed undi-
minished, his voice and his manner had grown much gen-
tler. When he spoke, the pain ceased. He examined me
without stethoscopes, reflex hammers, or electrocardio-
graphic leads. When he rested his head on my chest, I
could feel him listening to my heart and lungs, understanding all that which I had for so long found impossible

to say. He then ran his hands over my body, extracting each gossamer toxin that was a shadow of my form and dissolving it in a pool of sunlight. That is when I realized he was naked too, and that I was not ashamed of my urgent erection. Indeed, I felt a certain inexplicable power.

The door opened unexpectedly, putting a rather abrupt end to my dream. Then there was the clatter of a clipboard on a metal countertop, the cold stethoscope, the clumsy, almost punitive lubricated finger. I was given some intravenous fluid and, upon coming more to my senses, was given the diagnosis of a pulled intercostal muscle. Reassurance, it appeared, was the only medicine I needed. I returned to my dorm dumbfounded, and feeling more than a bit silly. It was only much later that I realized what had occurred in those few hours when I feared I was dying, even wished that I might die: I had located an intersection between my own mortality and the world around me, which was named desire. I wanted to live and to be loved, and at the same time I yearned to erase myself from the face of the earth. I wanted the morgue-like steel and chill of the doctor's office, and the warm hands of another upon my body telling me by their touch that I would endure.

Not long after this incident, I made love to my best friend for the first time, confirming what we had known for almost two years. What barrier it was that had been removed by my experience of illness, I could not have articulated then. I can report now, however, the healing I felt in each kiss, each touch, each murmured word. My body belonged to me again, as soon as I had owned its desire. To examine the crossing of this threshold—from bodily illness to mental health, from repressed misanthrope to unabashed queer—I changed my scientific methodology from neurophysiology to prosody, my tools from physics equations to rhyme, my materials from atoms to phonemes. If straight science could not provide the vocabulary I needed, perhaps the mysterious and complex human body could explain itself to me in its own terms.

It is through language, then, that I have found a way to love my patients, to desire them and thus put to work one of the most powerful elements of the therapeutic relationship. Present in my poetry is both the rhythm of my grandmother's praying and the thudding of a flashlight striking flesh. I am healing myself when I write, dancing close to another's body to a favorite Spanish song, allowing my mouth to find another man's mouth, because writing itself is the meeting of two expressive surfaces, that of the mind and that of the page. I can press my ear to my patients' chests in each lyric, and lie down for the long night beside them in each narrative. The pleasure in touching their skin I experience again in the pleasure my hand creates as it brushes against the smooth page. The love I feel for them is in the beating iambic heart of my lyrics.

The image of the page as yet unwritten upon conjures up powerfully an image of my patient Mary, smoothly bald and pale white from chemotherapy. On the bone marrow transplant unit, because most patients stay for such long periods of time, hospital rooms are transformed even more undeniably into their bedrooms; each morning I would visit Mary in hers during my rounds. Our encounters were always preceded by my ritualistic hand washing, obeying the strict rules to prevent infection, as the bone marrow ablation therapy she had undergone left her devoid of the cells responsible for immune function. She could not have been more naked, more available and accessible to others, more beautifully free. As I let the warm water run over my hands, I would begin to forget that soap I was using was bacteriocidal, as the killing of even the smallest of organisms seemed to have no place in our growing intimacy. I imagined at times that I was visiting a secret love, so much urgency did I feel in her desire to live. We spoke in hushed tones, hardly a word about the progress of her cell counts, more and more about silly, temporary things like our favorite Chinese restaurants, how much we each owed in parking tickets, the nurse's new butch haircut. On and on, like teenagers in a booth at a soda fountain. When I'd leave, I feared during the long hours I was away from her that I might never see her again. When I'd cry, she'd tell me to shut up. Wondering whether she felt the same way I did, I'd feel my heart quicken at the slightest intercourse: my ungainly otoscope whispering light in her ears, my slinky stethoscope hearing her heart's demand to live, my stiff penlight prompting the inexplicably delicious constriction of her pupils.

Many doctors must fall in love with their patients, though far, far fewer would likely dare admit it. What else were we to do, one of us dying less quickly than the other, the other less capable of preventing death than the first.

So we loved each other in the ways that we could. We listened to each other attentively and held hands. I write about her now, and she is alive. Constrained as we were by our respective worldly roles, as doctor and patient, gay Latino man and straight white woman, still we found the space to make a very particular kind of love—a love that concerned itself less with gender than with transcendence. Highly erotic and deeply pleasuring without our ever having slept together, as commonplace and yet unexpected as life crossing over to death, immortal as each retelling or the act of writing. Both Mary and I left our loving friendship healthier, I think, closer to being cured. She waved to me as she left the hospital, still bald, still beautiful, but more full of life, the life we shared.

However, I remain fearful for the future of this sort of honesty. The so-called personal lives of physicians and patients—as if the organs of emotion could be so carefully dissected in such an acute relationship—are already the subject of a scrutiny that seeks to eradicate the possibility of human connections. One needs to look no further than the cover of a major newsmagazine that appeared not too long ago to see the face of a physician so many now fear; ironically, though it was an image meant to sensationalize, it is a face as exquisite in its beauty to me as those of so many of my patients. The story was about a possibly homosexual dentist with AIDS who allegedly infected several of his patients with the virus, and who had died leaving behind a furor: *How did he give it to them?* the text of the article insistently asks.

I am certain that the hysteria around the issues of doctors with AIDS reflects at least in part the deep anxieties that come with recognizing the desire inherent in the patient-doctor relationship. Such fears remain pervasive in the culture at large, specifically with regard to the queerness inherent in a profession that in its practice crosses so many boundaries. Suddenly every lurking suspicion could be true, and each resentment is justified. The bespectacled, nerdy older man sticking his colonoscope up your ass actually *likes* it; worse yet, so might you. The image of sick physician as queer parallels the equation of AIDS = gay man. So it is not surprising that the same old sanitizing tactics have once again become implemented, with rules having been laid down as to which procedures are "safe" for HIV-positive physicians to perform and which are not—without a single shred of scientific evidence to suggest that the virus could even be transmitted through the contact such guidelines seek to limit.

People with AIDS, of course, were the subject of aggressive attempts at quarantine long before the public at large began to mistrust its physicians. Doctors themselves, it seems, could all too capably imagine the intimate contact they might have with their patients; the preexisting mechanisms for control present in the profession made it even easier for physicians to insulate themselves from people with AIDS under their care. During medical school I often overheard interns, residents, and attending physicians trying to guess which patients were most likely to give them AIDS through some vividly imagined mishap: the effeminate patient who squeals and jerks his arm away abruptly during a blood draw and thereby causes a needlestick, the normal-appearing hemophiliac who undergoes emergency surgery for appendicitis, the drug addict who vomits forcefully into the face of the rescuer performing chest compressions during an overdose-related cardiac arrest. In some cases, those patients known to have AIDS would receive less attentive care because of such fears. To this day, some surgeons outright refuse to operate on patients with AIDS, even on those they suspect might harbor the virus. Other physicians simply insist on proof of seronegativity before undertaking any invasive procedure.

As an new intern on the wards in San Francisco, I too fell prey to fears of AIDS, each emaciated body I encountered seeming a potential version of me. I saw my own face over and over again in their faces, the dark complexions, the mustaches, the self-deprecation. Incapable as I was then of loving my patients, I hated them instead for reminding me that I was no different, that despite my medical knowledge I was not invincible. My well-rehearsed internalized self-loathing dominated my emotional response to them. I wished that they would hurry up and finish dying, all of them in one fell swoop, and that they would take all the dying there was left in the world with them when they did. In time, my heart was gradually pressed out of me, and I blamed my inability to cry on the long, dehydrating hours I spent in the hospital. Instead of making love with my partner on the nights we shared a bed together, I slept fitfully, inhabiting personalized nightmares about AIDS.

In some ways, I know I have been dying of AIDS since the moment I first learned about the virus. Each smooth tube of blood I draw seems to come from my own scarred and indurated veins, each death note I have dictated has my own name and signature at the bottom of the page. Any disease that could erase from the world the bodies of so many people like me, people with whom I had not even had the chance to form the bonds of community, would seem necessarily to take with it small parts of my anatomy; AIDS has cut off the part of my tongue that once made it easy for me to sing, it has laser-ablated my seminal vesicles, it has occluded the blood flow to the area of my visual cortex capable of plainly seeing joy. What I had not been doing during those first few months of internship was trying to love despite the virus, or because of the virus. My healing powers, rudimentary as they were then, were hindered by a superficial wish to know death purely and simply as an enemy.

When I met Aurora, she changed everything. At first, she did not speak at all, except with her huge, moist eyes. I had admitted her to the hospital at 2 A.M. one grueling on-call night, with the emergency room diagnosis of "AIDS failure to thrive." (It was not until two weeks later that Aurora told me that she was dying of love, of too much love; cynically, I assumed she was referring to her own licentiousness.) Aurora was a preoperative male-to-female transsexual according to the terms of some of my colleagues; to others, she was a freak. My jittery and bumbling attending physician wondered with a nervous laugh on our formal rounds at her bedside the next morning what "it" had between "its" legs. Aurora just stared at him with her incredible eyes. I had written the order that she be placed in isolation, because her chest X ray was suspicious for tuberculosis. "Consumption," she would murmur to me later, "yes, I believe I am being consumed by my having loved too deeply." I was too busy to notice then the campy melodrama in her tone of voice; I could barely breathe through my protective fiberglass-mesh mask, and thought only of getting out of her room as soon as possible.

One day she began to flirt with me. "I know you're in there," she purred into my ear one morning as I mechanically examined her. I paused only briefly before I plugged my ears with my stethoscope, with the intention of listening to her heart sounds. Without saying anything, I raised her hospital gown up to her nipples, this time noticing the fullness of her breasts, the rich chocolate color of her nipples, the deep grooves between her delicate ribs. "Do you think I am beautiful?" She brought a crimson silk scarf up to her eyes and peered seductively over it at me. Her eyes were made up in three shades of green, the eyeliner and eyeshadow thickly applied. I had seen her at her mirror only once, hands trembling slightly, as she applied her cosmetics. At that moment I had thought her beautiful, not at all pathetic or threatening or "failing to thrive." She seemed hopeful and human, full of the love she kept so rapturously spilling out to those around her. But I was too busy to give much thought to what I had felt; my job was not to feel but to palpate. Not to love but to diagnose.

During the course of about eight weeks, Aurora gradually deteriorated despite the intravenous fluids and antibiotics. Her cough became more insistent, as though it were
finally winning a long, drawn-out argument. She appeared
less frequently in her flowing emerald green kimono and
stopped putting on her eye makeup. She gossiped less
about the other patients and no longer held court in the
patient lounge, where she had often been seen pointing out
the cute male passersby with her nail file as she manicured
herself. I pretended not to see her; I still listened only to her
heart sounds and not to her heart. "You know you're gonna
be mine," she sang out to me on another day in her naugh-
tiest Spanish Harlem accent, parodying one of the day's
popular dance club songs. I rolled my eyes as I left her
room. I never said more than a few words to her on my visits. I busied myself instead with collecting the data of her
decline: the falling weight, the diminishing oxygen satura-
tion readings, the recurring fevers. "I'm burning for you,
honey," she said with arched eyebrows by way of good-bye
on the last day she spoke. Again I said nothing.

Expecting her usual chatter more than I ever could have
admitted, I strode into her room the next morning without
knocking, as was my habit. No salacious remark greeted
me, however, no invitation to sit close to her on her bed,
no perfume. The silence registered. She seemed to be
lying sideways in her bed, with her face half-buried in a
pillow. The room's curtains had not been drawn open yet;
she remained motionless as I jolted them apart, flooding
the bed with sunlight. I glowered impatiently at her from

the bedside; still, she did not move. When I rolled her over, seeing her face stripped of all her glittery makeup, expressing not recognition but a deeply subterraneous pain, a primitive and wordless agony, finally I was moved. As I groped for her, finding her body half-paralyzed and oddly limp and angular like a bird that has flown into a windowpane, I began to feel broken myself. I was witnessing the loss of love from the world. Finally in its absence I was hearing her voice, and when I frantically listened to her heart and to her lungs for the first and last time I heard the love in them. I heard my own stifled desire surface for air in my long sobs.

Aurora died later that day, and when she died she left behind an element of herself in me. I find her voice in mine, like a lover's fingers running through my hair; my voice sounds warmer, more comfortable to me now. I discover her hands on my own body when I examine a person with cancer, or AIDS, searching for the same familiar human landmarks that bespeak physical longing and intimacy. Her glorious eyes return to me when I finally see someone for the first time, or when my own bring forth tears. Her friendship and her love of life return to the world in these words, in the poems I write that I hope might ascend to reach her in whatever realm she may now exist. Instead of giving me AIDS as I had so irrationally feared, she gave me hope.

Science failed to understand her, though it altered her body. Medicine did not love her, though it penetrated her with needles and X rays. Only the act of writing can find her now, because it is the same journey she has made, from the imagined to the actual, from the transitory to the persistent. From the unspoken to this physical and loving lament.

Like a Prayer ~

*Then, as a studious adult, I was confirmed in my training and vocation
by the credible narratives of the four gospels and the specific and implied
ethic of Jesus (though I reserve my assent to some other texts of the
Christian Bible). The miraculous events of his life are reported in a
straightforward manner that compel my belief—above all, in the fact of
his healing power and his bodily resurrection from the tomb.*
       —Reynolds Price, from "At the Heart"

    Only the inmate does not correspond:
God, lover of souls, swaying considerate scales,
Complete thy creature dear O where it fails,
    Being mighty a master, being a father and fond.
       —Gerard Manley Hopkins, from "In the Valley of the Elwy"

As I went about inattentively jotting down his
vital signs, and then taking a perfunctory listen to his
heart, he entreated me with a voice so raspy from disuse
it was almost gentle: "Hey, doc, when you get to church
this morning, pray for me." A few soundless moments
passed. After I had said nothing in response, he added
with the same hoarseness that at higher volume became
a surprisingly vicious snarl, "Yeah, you must be a real
good fucking Catholic, with a name like that." Now I was
annoyed, to have been startled out of my dim reverie,
and by such a crass slur. Was he referring to the Latino-

voweled surname blazoned on my plastic ID tag, I wondered—or perhaps, I thought with rising contempt, he
was familiar with the lesser-known archangel Rafael?

I had simply been trying to get through my tedious
daily morning work rounds without a hitch, the hypnotic
lines of Madonna's latest hit song, which I had blasted on
my car stereo on the way to the county hospital, still pulsing suggestively over and over again in my head: *"Just like a
prayer / your voice can take me there / just like a muse to me / you are
a mystery . . . "* For the whole of the twenty-minute drive in
to work that day, I had kept my car's front windows rolled
all the way down to let the bracing wind and all of frivo-
lously sun-drenched San Francisco pour unimpeded into
me as I sped down Potrero. But the deepening poverty was
too obvious to ignore, the Mission district looking more
and more like a destitute Latin American country with
each passing block. As a last resort, I tried to make myself
admire a few colorfully attired hookers still working their
street corners at 6 A.M., the dawn for them meaning not
the beginning but the end of yet another day. Anything to
bring me outside of myself to some kind of an awakening,
to shock me into feeling more a part of the kingdom of the
not dying.

I had not even realized that the gorgeous day I wanted
so desperately to relish was a Sunday. For me, a dysfunc-
tional intern stumbling through my last in-patient rotation
with only randomly and infrequently scheduled days off,
each day had grown monotonously more and more indistinguishable from the one before it. Death was inevitable

and omnipresent; resurrection was not only impossible but ludicrous. The hushed and somber hospital, whose hermetically sealed neighborhoods of illness and contagion went in house staff parlance by various quasi-celestial nicknames—the busy cancer unit was sarcastically referred to as the Death Star, and the grim and even more crowded AIDS ward was known as the Temple of Doom—had long been my exclusive place of dark worship and forced atonement. If I would have preferred to be in church, it was only because I so despised the hospital.

His nurse entered with a gelatinously floppy bag of IV fluid to hang. According to her, my patient had been babbling incoherently off and on for much of the night, yet I felt how unmistakably and clearly these last few words of his pierced me. *Pray for him?* This patient was a filthy junkie who had bitten another nurse in a squabble over his regular methadone dose; numerous times, I had been paged in the middle of the night and awakened from a precious hour or two of sleep to respond to his incessant demands for other narcotic drugs to treat his "pain," always to arrive to find him resting in apparent comfort amid half-emptied take-out cartons of Chinese food brought in by his rowdy, ponytailed friends. If I could have hoped or prayed for anything, it would have been that he'd be stone-cold dead when I next returned to the ward.

Instead, to my chagrin, each morning he was still there, very much alive and moaning and urinating in his bed, or hurling the occasional intelligible and angry epithet at me. Though nothing was likely to salvage him at this point in his illness, with his terminally low T-cell count of 2, a long history of violence and intravenous drug use, and widespread aggressive lymphoma involving his central nervous system, I was still leery of trying anything new at all—even a begrudged prayer—that might prolong his misery, and thus my own. He was little more than a disgusting chore to me, something akin to mopping up a stubbornly grimy floor. In my view, each new hospitalization he had required, thickening his chart as if only to make it heavier for me to lug back and forth from medical records, was a waste of already scarce public health dollars. This latest crude remark of his was the last straw. I stormed out of his room without even bothering to finish examining him.

By simply going elsewhere in the hospital, however, I could not escape him. I saw versions of him shadily averting their eyes in the elevator, hungrily consuming free food provided by the methadone clinic in the cafeteria, and wildly quarreling in the outdoors smoking area off one of the hospital's main hallways. Wherever I looked, his blunt plea would flood back to me, only to elicit the same reflexive rage. Though one of my intern's strategies for conserving energy was to minimize thinking whenever possible, I found myself obsessively wondering whether I walked around stooped by the heavy burden of some unresolved religious guilt, so that even my most ostensibly faithless and disoriented patients could tell that I was once a Catholic. My hip Ray Ban sunglasses, my pumping Madonna CDs, my chilling surliness, even my Gay Pride T-shirts worn secretly underneath my scrubs all failed to secularize me sufficiently in the discerning eyes of others. Even through the thick fog of his delirium, somehow he had alighted upon my name.

My name. I locked myself in a windowless staff bathroom, the only place I could think of where I could be completely alone, if the pungent presence of ammonia were ignored. I wondered: What secrets did a name betray? I regarded it from a distance as if for the first time, quietly pronouncing it over and over to myself; undeniably, "Rafael Campo" was as generically Latino as a colorful street festival for a local miracle-working Virgin, but my actual relationship to the Catholic Church was much cooler than my stereotypically churchgoing family's. I was a hard-core outcast for my supposedly sinful life, and no longer even considered myself a member of any faith. It amazed me that a low-life like this patient, who probably had stolen stereos from cars in the hospital staff's parking lot to pay for the heroin he was known to shoot directly into his IVs, could still consider himself among God's children, worthy of a saving prayer.

After all, "Mary" had to my snide and deconstructed ears become merely slang for a gay man, no longer the sacred name of the Virgin Mother of God, while "Jesus" was one of the greasy Mexican hospital janitors' names, or a cheap expletive, a rather meek expression of exasperation or anger. Yet I had been insulted by the derision in his voice, as if certain elements of my religious upbringing still bound my heart, still commanded my affections. That he so easily prompted me to rise up and *defend* my latent

Catholicism, challenging me to define myself more clearly, made me all the more furious.

Much as I hated being pigeonholed, and erroneously at that, I loathed him most of all for what I presumed was his very desire for absolution. What impudence entitled him to ask for forgiveness, I fumed, when I myself dared not pray for anything anymore? What made him believe he even needed to be forgiven? My own crisis of faith had gone far beyond what seemed in my jadedness and self-absorption the routine, even knee-jerk questioning of the existence of an omnipotent and benevolent God in an abstract world where millions of children are homeless or abused, where millions more innocent people are killed, raped, and tortured each year, where countless patients die every day despite all the heroic interventions of modern medicine—in the same world where, it seemed, much more outrage could be provoked when a crumbling old church was converted tastefully into architecturally unusual condos, or a photograph of a crucifix immersed in urine was called art. I had seen dazed elderly people brought into the ER covered in their own shit, gaunt children with the imprints of irons burned into their soft skin. The real atrocities of the world had become commonplace and automatic for me, to be relived every time I entered a hospital, not merely pondered in the lofty contexts of metaphysics or politely debated in the more banal arena of social policy.

I just could not be bothered with the plight of others anymore, on any level. As if to protect myself, I focused on the many injustices I felt so acutely in my own life. I had allowed myself to become deeply concerned that my own great potential had been blighted by that one imponderable aspect of myself that I never had wished for or willfully chosen. I was, I had realized long ago, among the not blessed. (Some would say, as I once heard on a religious radio talk show, that I was being used unknowingly by Satan himself!) I imagined my elderly Latina patients cursing me with a serpent's hiss—*maldito seas*—if they were ever to discover my vice. I was an abomination to the same God they said had created me, and whose forgiveness at the same time was the only hope for my salvation. When I tried to conceive of the possibility of redemption, I felt my flesh tearing, my bones popping mutely out of their sockets, my wretchedly human body unable to stretch across the rift growing between me and the withdrawing heavens toward which I reached out. It was the kind of fracture that all my years of medical training would never be able to repair. A queer still desiring and perhaps even needing some form of a relationship with God, I bitterly embodied as deep a schism as any in the Catholic Church's long divisive and blood-soaked history.

So what "prayer" would a misfit like me intone for the likes of him, anyway? Despite my well-groomed hatred and my practiced efforts at execration and denial, I had to admit that I did recognize him. He was my brother, another human being, just as pathetic and frightened, just as despicable and unforgivable as I, and asking for the same soothing words I both craved and actively refused. Even so, he remained as hideous to me as I believed myself to be to my estranged Catholic faith, and so by a strange arithmetic he was unsuitable as the subject for any form of art, even mine. If I had any religion left in me at all, it was only a distorted reflection of Catholicism, it was the potential for frenzied creation that arises from abjection and loss mixed with a brutally repressed hope of reconciliation. My "visions," my poems, contained some amorphous, nascent, not-too-ugly shapes, demanding to exist in spite of what I considered to be their ultimate valuelessness. For me to become a healer and a poet, a healer through the unabashed writing of poetry, seemed an unattainable dream, something that could occur only if Christ would somehow agree to appear less radiant and noble in his suffering than all of the masterpieces of the Renaissance had depicted him.

Or perhaps, I often thought, if only I could find the right place to begin. But Adam was always fucking Steve in my stunted garden of Eden; my pitiful pidgin language would always consist only of the words left out of prayers. Certainly, I would always be Catholic to the extent that I could accept what I did not understand as a kind of mystery, from the workings of the body whose interior was as dimly and creepily illuminated as a medieval cathedral's dank reliquary, to the creation of the sibilant voice with its unbounded capacity for healing despite its unimpressive anatomical dimensions. Still, I recalled another face of Catholicism, which decreed that certain things in the world were categorically unacceptable, far less mysterious than they were frankly vile. In the attacks of so many hateful sermons, in the misinformation propagated by so many Catholic thinkers, my enforced and obligatory corruption and its attendant rage had accumulated in me over so many years that at the time it seemed impossible for me ever to reconnect. I was so resigned to what was called my sin, it had become my grinning muse and corrupted master, my terrible fate.

Of course, I remembered learning about other so-called sins as a child in Sunday school; they seemed carefully choreographed and intentionally committed, in contrast to the way my heart spontaneously quickened and lurched with a music my teachers said was abhorrent and unnatural. Adultery, moneylending, and the like seemed somehow more egregious and deliberate than what had been born into me. Yet while at least half of my playmates' investment-banker parents seemed to have been divorced simply because they could not get along, and the blatant two-timers among the other half kept their nice jobs (and usually their nice families), homosexuals were summarily fired, punished, blackmailed, disowned, or beaten to death in back alleys. (It was always the home of the two faceless men who lived together in my neighborhood that the older kids pelted with eggs and draped with toilet paper, their mailbox the one they blew up regularly with firecrackers.) Even the sleaziest of prostitutes and the most recalcitrant of thieves could be pitied and so could redeem themselves in the judgmental eyes of the faithful; the examples of Mary Magdalene and Judas proved it. But

there was no conceivable rehabilitation for queers, no biblical provision for anything besides their anonymous,
incendiary, and sulfurous Old Testament destruction—
which was partly what I supposed kept them out of the
Church, cowering in their closets, or suffering in hospitals.

"Homosexual" seemed far too extreme a word for what I
might be, anyway; I had a family that loved me dearly, no
matter what, and a merciful Church that held me close to
its pounding heart. I could still recall when I had been
quite snug in the arms of my accepting, vibrantly religious
culture, before the revelations and the accusations, before
the realization and rhetoric and rejection. The Church
warmly stoked the fires of my imagination; the Church was
a far grander family home, the priest a more distant but also
more patient and forgiving father. The Church was a sanctuary in times of war; I imagined members of my family
hiding out safely behind the thick doors of dusty old
cathedrals in Cuba as the revolution swirled malevolently
around them. The Church was also a place of healing, the
prim nuns doubling as equally prim nurses, the pews
cleared away to make room for wounded soldiers on their
stretchers.

The Church was also a form of restitution. Very little in
my childhood surroundings truly belonged to me in suburban New Jersey, where there were few Cubans, or even
Italians, but in a Catholic church I was on the inside of all
creation, the meek inheritor of a vast earth; inside its
unmovable, inviolable walls, I was so secure that I felt the
polished wood and hard marble as if with my exposed

heart pressed to their cool, smooth surfaces. A Catholic church represented all the awesome power of conquering Spain and merchant Italy, all the accumulated, bygone strength of my faceless ancestors. Inside the fortress of my beliefs, like a milky pearl inside the rough oyster's shell, I had echoing words that mollified and contained those concepts too frightening to imagine without them, I had prayers that gave resplendence and structure to what I ardently believed, and I had solid-gold dogma to organize the world tangibly and hierarchically into good and evil. The bits of Latin uttered solemnly during mass were so much like Spanish that they implied that even my possibly shameful ethnic heritage was fit to be set to ethereal music. Poetic language began for me upon a praying priest's lips, in the rhythmically intoned words that seemed as luxurious and sensually attractive as his flowing gowns, in the perfect music of impossibly strict rules. In the unsayable name of God and His first regally alliterative, choriambic command: Let there be light.

More than its gritty mortar and glowing icons, more than what it could give physically to me, the Church itself was a vessel brimming literally to its spires with symbolic and mysterious poetry. Poetry flowed in the supple warmth of votive candles lit by the trembling hands of supplicants, whose soft voices mixed with the tenuous light thrown across the highest rafters. Poetry blinded whole congregations in the gleam of the silver chalice raised for God's most precise inspection. The comforting word was present even in the worn and faded velvet lining of the offerings basket, which looked as if it might also serve as a cozy resting place for the neighborhood's stray cats that the priests took in. Any creature was welcome in my romanticized, hymn-drenched Catholic Church— even the most irretrievably lost of wanton souls. And anything could be imagined with a heartfelt prayer.

A prayer was much more, however, than its reverent, richly structured language; a prayer was human word steeped in divine power. A prayer evoked the desiring mouths and lungs of centuries upon centuries of believers, of celibate priests and nuns who loved only Christ and the Church. A prayer was forgiveness, and as such a prayer was healing. We prayed for the sick members of the parish, our united, gently reverberating voices even more comforting than the quilts stitched by the hands of a hundred women parishioners. With prayer, Jesus revived the dead Lazarus, literally breathing life back into him; a prayer was what we murmured at the gaping graveside, when all the medicine in the world had finally failed. A prayer was the catalyst for miracles, the unthinkable transubstantiation of bread and wine into the body and blood of Christ. A prayer was universal. Whether my family prayed in English or in Spanish, it strangely sounded the same, reassuringly meditative, humming, penitent, restrained; we prayed in New Jersey the same prayers offered in far-off Cuba. Most of all, a prayer was love, an expression of God working through the imperfect but irresistible mortal body, moving the priest's heart, opening it and closing it as smoothly as the red-and-white satin he wore as he blessed us. A prayer was nothing less than an incomparable, inexhaustible, incontrovertible poem.

As I grew older, however, I wanted more. I wanted to curl up against the fantastic warmth of a miracle, I wanted to touch the full, adoring lips that gave shape to those sublime words, I wanted to taste the fingers that placed the dry wafer to dissolve on my tongue, I wanted to swim in the red-and-white satin that the priests wore; meanwhile, Sunday school was devoted more and more to warnings about our maturing bodies. I began to dread having to attend classes, because I was certain the nuns and priests knew something about me, something awful, something sinful. But I was not yet sure exactly what it might be. If anything, perhaps I loved Jesus too much; I drew countless pictures of his handsome face, of his nearly naked body on the crucifix or standing transfigured on the peaks of unidentified mountains, and kept them hidden in my desk drawers. To my growing distress, each church wedding I attended united a man and a woman in holy matrimony, and at the youth group dances to which my parents forced me to go, boys danced only with girls. The priests who lived together in the rectory were married to the Church, and not to each other, my parents explained in response to my persistent questioning; still, there seemed no practical way for *me* to be with another man. Each night, I prayed to the God whose only son had died for my sins to give me what I wanted most of all: an explanation of what hurt, a reason for why I too wanted to die.

Then, one Sunday during mass, my mind adrift in the

sea of colorful light filtering down from the stained glass
window above as I recited the Apostles' Creed, I made the
inconceivable and irrevocable connection, felt the blazing
brand of recognition—as if I had finally been given the gift
of life, been filled almost unbearably by what I could only
identify as the Holy Spirit: *I* was the degenerate homosexual whom I imagined my Church so despised. I felt I had
been chosen and, in the same excruciating moment, oblit-
erated. Suddenly everything made perfect sense to me, and
yet was all the more terribly incomprehensible. I recalled
that was how one of the younger priests in the parish had
once attempted to describe *faith*—unintelligible, yet
unquestionably true—but found no comfort in his words. If
it was a kind of faith that had seized me, it was in an entirely new religion. The kaleidoscopic light from above was
becoming the sacrilegious glitter of the gay discotheque I
had seen in movies, the angels were becoming beautiful
winged men, the prayer on my tongue tasted exotically
seductive. The power of prayer had worked again, but also
seemed cruelly to have failed me.

My transformation that morning was certainly not
conventionally miraculous, but I felt the astonishing repercussions at the core of my being as much as if I had manifested the stigmata on my hands and feet. Clearly this
horrible benefaction from my creator was to be my test in
this life, my sexy crown of sharp thorns to wear. Around
me, however, no one seemed to have noticed any change
in me at all. I exhibited no new shocking and inexplicable
powers. I healed no one, though surely I felt in my break-

ing heart an early stirring of the impulse to heal; I could speak neither to animals nor to God, but I soon wrote my first deliberate poem. After several months of soul-searching, when the time came for my confirmation in the Catholic faith, I resolved to confess to our parish priest what had been revealed to me about myself. I believed that what I contained was sinful, though it felt undeniably natural and wondrous, and I knew it to be a mysterious gift from God. I hoped that by confessing, and through the subsequent anointment into manhood, I would be restored to what everyone around me considered normal: that either this mistake would be remedied or that the world itself would just as miraculously change.

My day of reckoning came soon enough. My fall from grace was foreshadowed by the name I had chosen for my confirmation name: it was Michael, partly because of an innocent crush I had developed on a favorite aunt's new fiancé. As I came to the head of the line to receive the sacrament, surrounded by my giggling fellow catechists, my well-rehearsed lines stuck in my throat, as if in all my praying to God to make me like everyone else I had swallowed and choked on my precious rosary. I resigned myself to my fate the moment I entered that narrow booth; I confessed only to the milk-toast sins of fighting with my brothers and with my parents, and of being too selfish. The young priest who must have known I was different, who must have guessed at my inner spiritual turmoil, nonetheless quietly absolved me of *all* my sins, with no further discussion. I silently prayed that if God really existed, I would leave the confessional a different man. It would be my last request, I later realized, as a Catholic in good standing in the Church. When I stepped out into the steadfastly mute universe, greeted primarily by a sense of my own isolation and insignificance, I knew I was indeed changed.

Of course, the Church itself had not changed—it seemed just as incapable as ever of adjusting to the modern world—and I was impatient and sullen. I continued to go to mass for only as long as my parents could use guilt to motivate my attendance; I slept late on Sundays to avoid having to accompany them. Almost subconsciously, I began to find alternative means to cultivate the power I felt I could no longer savor in prayer. I wondered whether medicine might give me a similar power over life, and so a possible career took shape in my imagination. I also dabbled a bit more in poetry. I knew God worked through art, through the inspired images of the likes of Michelangelo, El Greco, and Leonardo, and I remembered how Christ himself had healed with words. The religious magazines that came to our house full of simpleminded rhyming devotional verse were oddly comforting, a gross approximation of the sounds I wanted to hear and to produce.

In the meantime the Catholic Church did nothing to stop my straying from the flock. With the increasingly conservative bent of the new pope, it seemed that no argument, no rational discourse could ever be initiated between me and what I perceived as so monolithic an institution, even if I could have been emboldened to speak out. There seemed to be no other recourse except to acquiesce to my exclusion. If there were others within its secret interior spaces whose voices could have been heard, who could somehow have influenced Catholic thinking as regards homosexuality, they were unknown to me, and I would have disputed their existence; as I gradually relinquished what had been one of the greatest comforts in my life, one of the first things I forfeited was my capacity for believing in miracles. I was just sixteen years old. One day, with hardly a hesitation, I gave to my sister the shiny gold crucifix I had always worn faithfully around my neck. It felt like giving away a part of my body, like a heart valve or an eyelid or a small muscle in my hand.

Because of the obvious and apparently nonnegotiable antagonism between me and my church, my youthful self-deprogramming at least superficially seemed an effortless and straightforward process. The place specificity of "Roman" superimposed upon the universality of "Catholic" had always puzzled me, to begin with; I had always wondered whether elsewhere in God's universe there were other, less restrictively qualified Catholics. During medical school I briefly but seriously considered converting to Judaism (motivated in part by an overeager and newfound identification with the history of persecution suffered by Jews, and in part by my admiration for the interrogatory tradition of rabbinical scholarship). Afterward, I halfheartedly staked out my spiritual camp on the nebulous terrain somewhere between what might be called atheism and secular humanism. No fire and brimstone rained down upon me, and I supposed as a nonbeliever I ought not to have expected any. I still thought I could see the beauty in the world, or at least a reassuring Hallmark version of it— in the constellation of fallen yellow stars beneath an autumn maple, in the giggles and shouts of bustling schoolchildren crossing a street beneath the protective watch of a crossing guard, in the way all of spring was carried on the shoulders of even the smallest sprouting plants, and even in the chorus of reverent voices that spilled out from one or another church I might pass on my way, always, to someplace else.

Ironically, at the same time I began to live up more and more to my avenging confirmation namesake: the further away I drifted from Catholicism, the more punishing (though wingless) an angel I became. As I grappled with the moral issues I faced from what I believed was my new bold perspective of a rational and free thinker, my "rational" judgment of others grew harsh and unfair because I felt myself to have been harshly and unfairly judged. Medical school and residency, those monuments to dispassionate Science, turned out to be the perfect arenas to hone the blade of my discriminating sword. By the time I became an intern, I sorely missed the healing power of prayer in my life; its last traces had been washed away when a good friend in whom I had confided the truth about my homosexuality nervously responded by promising she would pray for me. Suddenly, I realized with a weird finality that I was in no position myself to offer prayers, but instead was forever destined to be the object of others' charitable intentions, if I was lucky enough to escape their rancor. The direct line to a higher power was thus disconnected for me, and I was banished to live in a house without lights (but with all the other modern conveniences), a frustrated missionary on the dark, unholy outskirts of God's luminous city.

So my hateful IV drug-abusing patient became only the latest in a long series of people upon whom I defensively practiced my own belittling brand of hypocrisy. I had quickly and easily relegated him to the category of all those for whom aggressive state-of-the-art medical care is so truly futile it becomes distasteful: the elderly demented and abandoned patient with aspiration pneumonia or urosepsis intubated and receiving vasopressors and antibiotics intravenously in the ICU, the young woman with widely metastatic ovarian cancer receiving yet another round of toxic chemotherapy, the heart transplant candidate in the CCU on intravenous benzodiazepine and inotropic therapy who will never get a heart, because of active alcohol abuse, the crack-dealing patient undergoing his third emergency surgery to repair another lacerated internal organ after his seventh gunshot wound. Each bone marrow biopsy, each rectal exam, each electrocardioversion I performed seemed only to compound the indignity of it all. I watched with detachment at the end of so many lives, as unmoved and bored as if I were taking out the garbage. In the cold glare of my new secular reasoning, without their humanity, without even their souls, such patients became unmissable targets for the senseless blame I had once felt and now deflected onto others.

AIDS seemed to be the realm where I always felt most acutely the daily lack of miracles, the active deprivation of God's grace. It was also among AIDS patients that I saw most clearly my comfortable disengagement from humanity. So many of my AIDS patients had been cast out of their own religious communities and repudiated by their families, left to suffer and to die alone. To combat my impulse, whenever sense failed me, to turn back toward the musical restoratives of prayer and poetry, I frequently reminded myself that I was not among them, that I was somehow different. Internally I accused them of a quasi-religious checklist of crimes of which I believed myself to be innocent. They were promiscuous, while I was monogamous. They were stupid, stupid enough to get infected, while I was clever. They were fornicators, while I loved another man. They were failures; I, a young graduate of Amherst College and Harvard Medical School, was at a pinnacle of achievement and still full of promise. They fretted about the fates of their souls, while I knew there was nothing after this life. They would allow themselves to be judged by God, while I judged them haughtily.

Even as I rejected my fundamental human bond with such patients, I marveled at how my new gay brethren seemed to create an imaginary church of their own out of the oftentimes hostile outside world. The darkly drafty three-level nightclub evoked the cavernous internal space of the cathedral, campy Abba anthems were substituted for solemn hymns, and the priests' satin robes became the sequined dresses of drag queens. Though I knew few other gay people personally, I was surprised at how many of us there seemed to be, and astounded at how many apparently retained a faith in God. I read about how some celebrated commitment ceremonies with their families, taking vows before ordained ministers, while others volunteered for Catholic charities for people with AIDS. Some worshiped in thriving Unitarian or Universalist churches; the die-hard Catholics joined Dignity, the gay Catholic organization, and worshiped in church basements until they were barred even from those dingy, fluorescently lit spaces.

Eventually, I simply pitied other gay people for not seeing the hopelessness of what I considered to be some unwitting form of penance. Did they not recognize the enemy when they saw him? At my first Gay Pride march in New York City, religious protesters carried placards saying AIDS was our punishment from God, average-looking middle-aged white men and women angrily screaming "God hates faggots!" as we made our way past Saint Patrick's Cathedral. They were not overtly crazy, like the disheveled proselytizers I had seen often on city street corners ceaselessly proclaiming that the end was near; some of them had children, cute little girls in frilly pink dresses and scruffy little boys in Yankees T-shirts. The inspiring, uplifting beauty of the structure in the background only amplified the brutality of their words; the calmly blank faces of their children, all too ready to be written upon beneath the scrawled placards, were being inscribed with the same words. Since then, I have never been able to look again at a church, that once familiar and beloved sanctuary, without feeling a reverberation of that moment's dire fear—not so much that the demonstrators might have physically harmed me, but that they might be just as human and as angry as I am. That I might have been them, that I might be like them.

At the time, having found barely enough courage to make love with another man, I could never have aspired to, or even imagined, such wickedness as they attributed to me. I actually felt terribly unworthy of their venom, inadequately sex-crazed, only twenty-five years old and still full of wonder at the possibility of realizing, finally, what I thought I had been taught (in the same Sunday school class where I had first learned to loathe myself) was God's gift to all people: the fullest expression of love with another human being.

Naively—or perhaps wishfully—even when faced with such adversity, I could still get caught up in moments when I hoped I could be an instrument for God's work— even though I was no longer Catholic, even though I would labor outside the walls of the blessed domain, I believed that somehow God knew I was good and forgave me. Though I might deny it, I harbored the slim hope that I might still be saved, by helping to heal others and devoting my life to alleviating not simply the physical afflictions but also the spiritual ills of my patients. The consummation of my attraction to another man, and the painful journey I had made to the discovery of my deviant sexuality, I believed might only somehow deepen my empathy for the suffering men and women who would come to my office. I would be capable of understanding their feelings of betrayal, would be uniquely qualified to soothe their grief. But in reality it appeared my career was not turning out that way at all. When that despicable AIDS patient finally did die, seizing intractably and without my prayers, I was glad, and relished his death over an unappetizing late-night meal with a few of my colleagues in the nearly deserted cafeteria. Still I knew he would only be succeeded by others.

Sure enough, late one night on call a few days later, I was paged to place an IV in yet another patient with AIDS, one who belonged to an intern for whom I was cross-covering. He was an emaciated young man who was receiving wide-open fluid resuscitation for dehydration, until he pulled out his first catheter; his veins stood out beneath his yellow skin so clearly that they seemed to beckon me to enter them, so plump that my mouth even watered a little. I prided myself on my ability to obtain intravenous access, so at first I was only mildly annoyed that the nurse had called me to perform what appeared to be so easy a stick. She was probably overworked herself, though when I had arrived an hour or two after her page she seemed to be on a break, and this was one task that could be unquestioningly relegated to a defenseless intern, with the automatic, well-rehearsed apology: "I've tried three times, and I just can't get it."

In a few moments, I had gathered together the necessary supplies in a small heap at the side of his bed: a drape, some sterile gauze, a small syringe filled with saline, a bottle of iodine, a liter bag of normal saline and some clear coiled tubing, a few strips of tape, a rubber tourniquet, the flimsy but requisite pair of latex gloves, and a 16-gauge Angiocath. I had selected such a big needle partly to underscore to his coffee-sipping nurse, without having to say a word, how effortless the job would be for someone competent. The patient remained asleep while I set every- thing up, the arm I had selected dangling lifelessly off the side of the bed. When I tried to awaken him to explain what I was doing, before I said more than a few words he mumbled, "Just get it over with and get the hell out of my room." Unfazed, I accepted his gruff statement as informed consent and decided by way of retribution not to bother with lidocaine to numb the area. I positioned the gleaming needle at the bifurcation of an especially large vein, which was swollen nicely under the pressure of the tourniquet I had tightened while he still dozed.

As I applied traction with my other gloved hand above the puncture site, I watched intently as the needle pierced the skin delectably, anticipating with confidence the bright flash of red blood in the needle's small reservoir that would indicate that the lumen of the catheter was inside the vein. I marveled at the permission I had to inflict pain, to assault another person with a sharp object under the pretense that I was actually helping him, but knowing that he would be dead soon, just like the rest. I was more sur- prised than annoyed when no flash occurred; I was per- fectly positioned, and the vein was huge. I withdrew and made a second attempt, again with no success. Sweat began to trickle down my brow, and I had to hold his arm down forcefully with the same hand I was using to apply traction to the vein; he was moaning more and more loudly now. A purple hematoma was growing slowly under his skin where I must have nicked the vein, further unpleasant evidence that this was a sentient, living being I was working on, not just the cadaver I foresaw he would become. On the third pass, with my hands visibly trembling, I finally nailed it and, feeling more than a bit relieved, looked away for a moment. I needed to find the syringe I would use to withdraw blood and then flush in a small amount of saline to confirm the patency of my line.

Perhaps it was the strange violation, the unwanted communication of the outside world with so intimate an interior space that aroused him; perhaps it was the pain I knew I caused, but which I so callously, even sadistically, ignored as I focused on my task, that prompted him to react. Before I knew what had happened, he was sitting bolt upright, screaming at the top of his lungs and flailing his arms out in front of him, scattering my neat pile of materials across the floor. I tried to stop him. When the same needle pierced my own skin, my first thought was to deny the literal connection between us, one that emotionally I had been for so long incapable of accepting but that was suddenly as lasting as metal, as pointed as agony. Blood poured out of the hole in his skin so profusely that in seconds the left leg of my scrubs was soaked in it, and I felt the cool slickness against my thigh, perplexed that it did not feel warmer as it was absorbed. I finally came enough to my senses to call out for help and staggered to the door of his room, leaving sticky, bloody sneaker prints behind me, my path in life momentarily made visible by another's suffering.

The look of horror on the nurse's face pulled me across the remaining dimensions through which I had begun to drift, back into the real world. After we had together restrained him enough to apply pressure to the vein and control the bleeding, I went directly to the sink. Both gloves I wore were covered with quickly drying blood, and when I peeled them off, I noticed stonily that the one on my left hand had been pierced through. I washed my hands before looking at them and felt the sting of the anti-septic soap in the middle of the palm of my left hand, the same sinister hand I had used to hold down his arm, the awful hand that had felt the strain of his weakened muscles against me and then the needle's terrible bite. Still afraid to inspect the sore spot, I took my time patting my hands dry and unwillingly noticed flecks of blood on the crumpled white paper as I tossed the used towels in the trash. So I knew. My left hand balled in a fist, I calmly announced to the nurse that I was fine and that I needed to get changed into some clean scrubs, before I exited the room on wobbly legs; she seemed to hover above the dark pool of blood, plump and white and dumb as a dove, and the fact that she said nothing to me made me wonder if she suspected the truth.

The rent in my skin was only two or three millimeters in size, though the small amount of blood that had fanned out in the subcutaneous tissue made a dusky red spot that was alarmingly much bigger, maybe a centimeter or so. I squeezed out whatever blood I could, not knowing whether the drop or two I was able to express was mine or his, or mine mixed with his. I changed my scrub pants in one of the deserted hallways of the labyrinthine OR, the dried blood that had soaked in pulling at the hair on my thigh as I shucked them off, not caring if a stray orderly or scrub nurse happened to spy me undressed: I finally knew how human I was, I was made acutely aware in one terrible moment that all any of us has in the world is the same body. I wanted to pray that I had not been infected, I wanted to believe that a god, any god, had protected me. After I was changed, I found an open utility closet and shut myself in it with the syringes and plastic emesis basins and face masks and blue gauzy hairnets close around me. I stared into the wound in my palm beneath the dim yellow light from a bare bulb, my forsaken faith even more dim; I found that I kept thinking of Christ, with the incongruous and gruesome fact dancing in my mind that in Roman crucifixions the nails were driven not through the palms, as seen in conventional depictions of Christ on the cross, but through the wrists.

I recalled that I had once stuck myself with a needle a few years before, as an inexperienced medical student attempting to draw blood from another patient with AIDS, but that incident had left no mark in my skin, and I had found no hole in the gloves I was wearing. Still, I had been unable to sleep for weeks, and it was several more months before I could even talk about it with anyone. In contrast, what was happening to me in the utility closet felt like an opening, a revelation, a chance for survival; though I certainly would not report to the Needlestick Hotline what had happened to me, perhaps there would be someone else, some higher authority, who would listen to me. Perhaps in the mixing of my blood with another person's, I could learn the true meaning of forgiveness, I could understand human failings, I could begin to fathom how we all share original sin. Perhaps in the possibility of dying of AIDS myself, I could realize finally and fully my capacity for empathy. Perhaps in a prayer, in a poem, in an embrace and a kiss, I could speak again to God.

These days, my version of the physician's "God complex" is to pray secretly at the bedsides of my patients, sometimes thinking myself silly for doing it, but finding it impossible not to do so. Whatever my religion might be—Catholic or Doctor Not of Theology, Queer Sister of Perpetual Indulgence or Undecided—I understand now that one's faith is intensely personal, in the same way each individual has his own hopes and dreams, and that it can be shared not only within the thick walls of churches but also in the open wards of a hospital. In my visions now, the patients who are dying, or who are getting well, all have a place to go; each holds inside and is held by the beating heart and the feverish closeness of his loved ones. Even the most despised and isolated of patients has someone to whom he can turn, one who truly does have the power to heal, a hope that is the source of all poems. The terrifying needlestick is just a reminder, the bearded chaplain on his rounds exudes a kind of comfort, the hideous skin lesion becomes the glorious imprint of God's touch. Today I see that the handsome nurse carrying away feces in a bedpan is an angel; the quiet glance we exchange is the meaning of life.

The Fairiest
College ~

A would-be physician who knew next to nothing about healing, I tried to envision myself at Amherst College. Standing atop Memorial Hill, looking out over the patchwork quilt of athletic fields, forests, and farms that stretched before me all the way to the undulations of the Holyoke Range, I felt the wind comb back my hair, trying to neaten my appearance in the same way my mother had before my interview; my father had wiped roughly at the corners of my mouth with a handkerchief he had moistened with his own warm saliva. Autumn was in full regalia, the world ready to die again in its own never-ending battle with itself. It was my second visit to Amherst. During my first visit, the driving rain had kept us squinting through bleary windows streaked with rain, as squarely compressed as our suitcases inside the family Buick, only imagining this celebrated view from "the Fairest College," barely glimpsing what was to be my future.

Throughout our trip across New England, we pored greedily over some glib guide to colleges and universities, which assigned to each a certain number of symbols—little stars, dollar signs, and telephones, for overall quality and competitiveness, tuition cost, and social life, respectively—and it was my assignment to read aloud from the text, which made me terribly carsick. I found myself, however, becoming fixated on getting into a place with the highest total number of symbols, and so I tallied them up for each college we visited, usually as we pulled in to the campus for the first time. Not only did Amherst have among the highest total number of symbols, I calculated, but it also said specifically in the text that it was among the most competitive in terms of percentage of applicants accepted: just less than 20 percent, compared with 20 or 25 percent at places like Harvard, Swarthmore, Princeton, and Williams. Amherst, at least according to this consumer-friendly template of values, was unbeatable.

So from the very beginning of my contact with higher education, I wanted most the place that wanted me the least. I wanted to prove that I could be accepted anywhere, even by tiny, arch-conservative Amherst College, which had only recently "loosened" its admission policies to allow women to enter. Even though its social life received just a measly three telephone symbols (instead of the maximal five symbols Amherst received in the other categories), and though my perpetually antagonistic younger brothers renamed it "the Fairiest College" as soon as they sensed my serious interest in it, I could barely maintain my attention on the droning tours of the other schools we visited over the next couple of weeks. For the first time in my life, I knew what I wanted.

The particular attraction Amherst held for me was its fabled and extremely rigorous premed program. Almost everyone who applied to medical school from Amherst was admitted. A crusty, impersonal biology professor with connections at all the best medical schools headed the premedical advisory committee, and an innovative neuroscience concentration (with a daunting number of required lab courses) had been developed for the most hard-core of premeds. Virtuously, I proclaimed to my family that I was interested only in the most broad of liberal arts educations, but on a deeper level I was drawn to this definitive, unwavering career track, a clearly marked path to an unambiguous identity. I suppose that I loved the smug duplicity of the place even then: a renowned liberal arts college that efficiently produced doctors, and also lawyers and captains of industry, in alarmingly high numbers.

Of course, I was also familiar with the august heritage of poetry at the college, which presented the only real problem for me as I grew more and more enamored of Amherst. Emily Dickinson had spent her entire life cloistered in the

small New England town and was buried in a nearby ceme-
tery. Robert Frost had taught at the college for many years,
and the new library at the center of campus was named
after him. James Merrill had actually attended Amherst
College, and his family name was inscribed on several
plaques scattered about the place, oddly including the one
that named the science building, the foreboding structure
where I imagined spending most of my time. In order to
sustain this venerable poetic tradition, a generously
endowed visiting poet's chair had been established in the
Department of English, to attract eminent contemporary
poets to its classrooms.

Such reverence for poetry conflicted with my efforts to
convince myself of its insignificance. Though poetry
might try to seduce me with the most base and primitive
charms of its thudding rhythms and emotional chants, I
was actively resisting its pull, aspiring to elevate myself
instead to the diaphanous plane of Science. Medicine was
the real discipline, the way of the future, a growth industry that was creating new jobs; medicine was the gleaming
metal and white of bustling hospitals and productive laboratories, the high-voltage shock to the stalled chest, the
glossy drama worthy of television or the movies. Poetry, I
wanted to believe, was only the dusty old library, the mere
candlelight of the Romantics, the utterance of an ultimately powerless priest; poetry was quaint and antique, and
could never revolutionize our lives.

Unaware of these internal conflicts of mine, my parents
looked upon my newfound attraction with consternation,

which only heightened the intensity of my passion for Amherst. In our heated discussions about my future, which always seemed to bring out my father's usually well-concealed Spanish accent, I defended my selection on the basis of its intellectual rigor, its physical handsomeness, its guarantee of a respectable career, and the bank-like sense of security it emitted. I could have been describing the qualities of the lover I had decided I would never allow myself to meet. It did not matter to me in the least that not a single Hispanic or black person had been visible on our tour, that not a single name inscribed on the war memorial reminded me of my own. In fact, at the time I feared any association with such people, and I especially took notice if a raving homeless person in Philadelphia or New Haven had been dark-complexioned. I wanted pure white snow on the pine needles outside my dormitory window, not a smudged view of the grungy stuff I had seen plowed to the sides of the clamorous Harlem streets around Columbia. I wanted priggish Calvin Coolidge, not flamboyant John F. Kennedy; I wanted a college environment that was utterly dignified and by implication well controlled, not one where the student union's walls were plastered with notices for open-mike poetry readings and anti-apartheid demonstrations. Most of all, and in spite of myself, what I really wanted was for my parents to approve of my choice.

Eventually, I was able to convince my parents of the merits of Amherst, which in the end did strongly appeal to their instinctual overprotectiveness. Perhaps they hoped it was the one most sheltered place where my deviant sexuality just might remain repressed, if they sensed at all what I so painstakingly attempted to eradicate in myself. Amherst College, solidly muscular with its bulky red-brick buildings, hewed out from a perilous wilderness by the most pious of men, oddly fatherly in the afterglow of its all-male tradition, armed with science and merely decorated with poetry, we all supposed would keep me safely sequestered. When finally I filed my application as an early-decision applicant, the forsaken pile of brochures and partially filled-out triplicate forms from the other schools we had visited seemed to huddle at the corner of my desk, conspiring against me, knowing what I was really trying to do.

Consciously, I was trying not to be attracted to any of the robustly handsome college guys who populated the campuses I visited. I wanted to make my decision with my brain, and not my heart. Most specifically, I tried not to remember the immensely appealing student who led the tour at Yale, whose picture graced their application materials, which happened to be on the top of the stack. He was what I might have called disdainfully then "a bohemian type," with long curly hair and a relaxed, almost magical smile. A small triangle of dark curly chest hair was visible at his open shirt collar, which had drawn me to him in spite of myself.

We had talked about literature, and particularly our mutual interest in the formal poetry of Elizabeth Bishop and James Merrill, as I the whole time attempted to impress him by shoehorning words like "prosody" and "alliteration" into our small talk. He asked me amiably how long I would be staying in New Haven, and whether we could have coffee together before I left town. Later, near the end of our conversation, he mentioned casually that there was a very active gay and lesbian student group on campus and that it would be glad to send me some information. I acted appalled. I told him, abruptly and in my iciest voice, that he was greatly mistaken and that I had long ago decided not to apply to Yale at all, but my parents were forcing me to take the tour anyway. At Amherst, in contrast, the burly student who gave the tour sported a smirk, a severe crew cut, and a dapper striped tie and did not take the time to ask me any questions at all.

My father still brought up Harvard from time to time as the weeks passed ponderously, saying I should not turn my nose up at such a fine institution, especially if things did not work out with Amherst. He had convinced himself that the school had expressed an interest in me, after he spoke for a second time with the woman in charge of minority recruitment in its admissions office. Even across the wide ocean, and then through the dense jungles of Cuba, he had heard transmitted the great name of Harvard University and long had dreamed of sending his son there. Perhaps it epitomized for him success in the United States of America, an antidote to the unbearable displacement he felt from his homeland; if the endless beaches and lush rain forests of Cuba could no longer be his, then maybe he could replace these memories with the openness of mind and the elaborate panoply of ideas his beloved island

lacked. It was as if to camouflage our unspeakable dispos-
session that we drove around in our shiny American car to
investigate the Ivies, and lived in a middle-class suburb
where fingernails and manners and lawns were all carefully manicured; for my parents to mention while playing
bridge with their friends that I had been accepted by
Harvard seemed the logical next step in the relentless
process of our quiet assimilation.

Education itself was indeed so precious and sacred to
my family that each report card was read as intently as a
prayerbook, each diploma was framed and hung at the
altar of aspiration. It was more than merely the stamp of
approval on the passport admitting us to America; it was
an elaborate faith. According to this quasi-religion in
which I was raised, an ultracompetitive college was like the
Vatican, representing the highest attainment possible for
earthly mortals. Admittance to a prestigious professional
school was equivalent to canonization. To become a physician was like entering the heavenly host—it was redemp-
tive, a kind of immortality, and for the entire family. My
parents had themselves proudly attended Catholic
University, at a very great sacrifice for their own parents;
because they had met there, the university also became in
my mind the place to fall in love, to find the woman I
would marry and who would someday bear my children.

It was all the greater an outrage to my parents, then,
that some young people went to college secretly hoping to
separate from their families, eager to explore their new
freedom by experimenting with sex and learning about

Marxism and atheism, along the way abandoning their goals of becoming professionals. Even stately Amherst might have its share of dissolute tenured radicals, ready to seduce me. Who knew what inflammatory and dangerously sinful materials I might be required to read, what unpatriotic and corrupt ideas I might be forced to embrace? While my parents prayed desperately for their children's continued academic high achievement, I sensed that they remained conflicted about the possible consequences of our actual enlightenment. Ultimately, I knew in my heart that what they most wanted was for me to be safe and happy, to be an educated man, but these frightening concerns of theirs inevitably weighed on me.

Fortunately, because the alternative would have meant scurrying at the last moment to mail in my other neglected applications before their looming deadlines, I was soon informed by a terse letter that I had been admitted to Amherst. My future as a physician suddenly seemed assured. My mother beamed and immediately started making expensive long-distance calls to relatives, my father came home from work *early*, and my brothers rolled their eyes in disgust that I had gotten—yet again, in their assessment—what I wanted. After the initial commotion, we all went out to dinner to celebrate at the local Mexican chain restaurant where I was working dutifully as a busboy to save money for college. My parents bragged to everyone around us as we waited for our table, suburbanites they did not know, about my accomplishment, mistaking in our delirious joy Casa Maria for a bona fide Latino gathering place.

That night I was too thrilled to be mortified. After we were seated, my father, who often reminded us that he rarely drank alcohol, astonished us all by ordering a bright-red strawberry margarita. When it arrived, he held it aloft proudly in a toast to my success. All my own dreams seemed concentrated in that ridiculously top-heavy drink, extravagant and sweet and awkward and delicious and contrived yet trying to be genuine, all at once. While canned mariachi music wailed tamely and distantly from some unreachable, unimaginably happy island, I felt that I had finally found my own place, *my* private island, a securely isolated home of my own. My father then drank deeply and ceremoniously from his glass; it left a trace of coarse salt on his upper lip, and some of the frozen concoction dripped down the side of the glass. In that single gesture, I felt again, but more clearly than I had ever felt it before, how much I was a part of him, how internally I was held by him, and for the first time feared how fragile he might really be.

The ensuing months before I left for college flashed by; the uncomfortably scratchy tuxedo that I wore to my senior prom, indistinguishable from those rented by my friends, and the big jewel-like tears my parents shed at my graduation from high school are the only sharp memories I seem to have registered from that time. I am certain that summer must have been a period of extreme anxiety for me. I nervously bought new underwear and socks whose pristine whiteness signified the new beginning, a kind of virginity that at the same time was sexy and yearned to be violated.

My brothers say that I ignored them, enveloped in what they presumed was a trance-like state of narcissistic self-congratulation. My sister, only five years old at the time, says that I began recruiting her to my beloved Amherst even then (a pressure she says she has continued to endure as she nears the end of high school herself). Saying good-bye to my friends and to my girlfriend, driving down the Garden State Parkway to the Jersey shore with the car windows wide open, and trying on drunkenness for real at various graduation parties—the frightened teenager in the photographs my parents have saved might have done these things, but not a version of me that I can recall.

I finally left the confines of suburbia, and after the now familiar four-hour car ride I arrived at Amherst, but this time I was one of her own. I was already becoming someone else, a different person: the sun seemed a bit less out of reach. At the freshman orientation barbecue, my parents hovered over my shoulder, eagerly pointing out details in the scenery and in the architecture, or solicitously offering to get me more of the watered-down pink lemonade, all the time avoiding what was the inevitable good-bye. Huge fists of smoke from the grilling steaks curled and rose in the air, dramatically giving shape to the growing resentment that began to boil in my blood. I was too indignant about my own efforts at coolness being spoiled to acknowledge either the strain in my father's voice whenever he asked me a question or the film of tears in my mother's eyes when she studied the cornice at the top of a pillar.

My father had assigned himself the special responsibility of spotting potential friends for me in the crowd, which I found especially irritating because his criteria apparently were (1) that they be male, (2) that they have short hair, and, most important, (3) that they have a Spanish-sounding surname. This third criterion required him to approach each prospective candidate quite closely while staring at his chest as he tried to make out the lettering on his scrawled name tag. Pathetic, I thought; even as he had spurred me on to reach so high an echelon in American culture, still he searched for traces of his lost culture (one I was glad to be rid of) that somehow might root me.

After about twenty minutes of this behavior, I told him plainly that he was embarrassing me, and pleaded with him to stop. I desperately wanted to blend in; I was actually working at being nondescript. Just then he shouted, squinting, "Look over there! JOR-ge A-RRO-yo," enunciating the name clearly, rolling his r's beautifully, almost seductively. "Now *he* looks like a nice guy. Why don't you go introduce yourself to him, and find out whether he's in any of your premed classes?" That was when I glimpsed the name tag myself, pinned to a colorful plaid madras shirt. As he walked by, his face turned toward an attractive, chattering woman with thick blond frizzy hair who clung to his elbow, my father lunged to grab his shirtsleeve. I winced—yet he had not heard my father call out his name, and my father missed him by more than a few inches.

When I had collected myself enough to speak, my voice was quietly and coolly irate. I stated that I would not select my friends solely on the basis of their ethnicity or their pre-professional choices, that I wanted to form friendships on the basis of shared interests and *not* presuppositions, and that I would make a point of *not* meeting this Jorge Arroyo, and for that matter any other Latinos or premeds, precisely because he wanted me to do so. Looking utterly crestfallen, my father trailed off to get us some more lemonade, drained of all his vicarious excitement, not knowing that ten years later he would be telling this same story gleefully, almost triumphantly, taking the credit for first identifying the man with whom I have spent most of my adult life.

Jorge Arroyo had long since dissolved into the crowd by the time my parents and I drifted back to our trusty Buick, which was parked at an odd angle along with a few other stray station wagons and U-Haul vans on the main quad in front of my new home. Sated carnivores after a bloody meal—the steaks were served up a juicy medium-rare—we seemed ready to disband and to roam onward. I looked up at the sky, avoiding my parents' eyes, and felt astounded by the number of stars already visible, so soon after the sun's setting. My mind was full of them, like all the brilliant and ineffable things I always had wanted to say to my parents but never could. My mother smoothed her skirt; my father plunged his hands into his pockets. In the end, I was terribly sad to see them go, but no tears of mine intermingled with theirs. *Doctors never cry*, I said sternly to myself, reminding myself why I had come to Amherst. My mother left a smudge of pink lipstick on my cheek, while my father folded a fifty-dollar bill and pressed it into my palm, "for emergencies." Then they were gone. I watched impassively as the Buick loped awkwardly and unevenly across the quad, and then heard the definitive slam of the back fender that scraped against the curb as they pulled out onto the road that would take them back to my old home.

If I felt at all sentimental, or if I feared a loss of containment in the wake of my parents' departure, I immediately found some reassurance in the up-front bigotry of my two roommates, both from upper-middle-class white families who lived in suburban New England. I was on my guard at once: "faggot" was among the first words they exchanged in casual conversation, as if to prove to one another, and to me, that it would be safe for us to sleep all three in the same room. It also seemed to be the only publicly acceptable derogatory term to name something as exotic as what I might turn out to be, with a weird name like Rafael; "spic" was clearly too impolite, too vulgar.

So it was that I began to feel the weight of the thousands of red bricks that surrounded me pressing upon my heart and upon my imagination, and it felt surprisingly good. Already I had guiltily noticed the bodies of some of my new male classmates as they unpacked, the bulges in the folds of their sweats catching my eyes involuntarily as I walked through the hallways of the fluorescently lit dorm, the beginnings of chest hair deliberately and proudly displayed beneath unbuttoned shirts. I was relieved, however, to find my own roommates much less physically appealing. As those first few weeks passed, even though the two of them were very different from what I had expected my new roommates to be like, and I knew in my disappointment I would never become their true friend, I felt strangely safe with them.

Since nothing about them tempted me, I could hang out with them and feel straight, trying to shore up what I began to fear might someday escape me entirely. One was bow-legged and short, with a thick, surly Boston-type accent; the other was taller and gangly, with a chronic sinusitis. Each, I soon learned, was a particular type of Amherst man: the drunken, frustrated, would-be athlete, and the snide, doped-up, directionless hipster. Their ceaseless fag jokes steeled me to the possibility of my own homosexuality, driving me during the daylight hours into the depths of my new biology and chemistry texts. Each was intent on proving his masculinity, always boasting his dick was biggest. In no time, and to my surprise, they developed a cadre of loyal fans. When one of them sent a woman from Mount Holyoke home clutching her blouse to her chest and crying from a blazing frat party, people laughed at her; when the other nearly scraped off his face after running into a tree while playing Frisbee stoned, people thought it was cool.

Frequent trips on the free shuttle bus (called the "fuck truck") to Mount Holyoke and Smith (where the women were all "dykes" because invariably, contrary to all reasonable expectations, they would not allow themselves to be screwed by such clearly desirable male specimens) often led to consummation instead in an inane rivalry with the

other main freshman dorm. On nights when my roommates had been locked out of one house party or another
at Smith or Mount Holyoke, they would return to
Amherst drunk and unsatisfied, and descend upon Stearns
Hall to remove the handles to the water faucets in the
shower stalls and on the sinks in their bathrooms, or clog
the toilets with toilet paper, or stop up the sinks and uri-
nate into them, or grease their doorknobs with Vaseline.
Then they would return to wait giggling in a state of near
ecstasy not only for the audibly indignant shouts to come
from Stearns the next morning but also to be "fucked over"
themselves in retribution. These encounters with the
enemy transpired on almost a weekly basis, with the
impressively erect, disembodied Stearns Tower—a tall
stone tower that was all that remained unscathed from an
old building that had burned down long ago—looking on
from its position behind both dorms with evident pleasure,
symbolizing the college's tolerance for, indeed enjoyment
of, this brand of male-to-male sexuality.

　Though I did not participate in these nocturnal activities,
fearful that they might fuel in me the urges I was already
fighting so hard to repress, I was curious about one thing in
Stearns Hall: whether Room 105 Stearns was as spacious as
my own, a much coveted two-room triple with a private
bathroom, Room 105 James. It had dawned upon me that
the dormitories were in fact enantiomers, mirror images of
one another like certain special molecules I was just beginning to learn about in Chemistry 11. Their external appearance was identical but opposite. So one day after class,

though it was contrary to all the rules about social associations set up by the warring factions, I entered Stearns in broad daylight with the intention of finding out who lived in Room 105. Turning to the left, instead of to the right as I would have done to reach my own doorway from the main entrance into James, I had the distinct sense that what I was doing was terribly wrong. I was crossing an inviolable threshold, and the world I discovered was entirely backward though absolutely familiar. The doors themselves were made of the same dark wood, but their frames were painted institutional red instead of institutional blue. Though hanging upon them were the same types of erasable message boards with their dangling Magic Markers, the handwriting and names and messages were all eerily different. Finally, my heart pounding wildly, I reached my destination. The "105" gleaming above the doorway before which I stopped was identical to mine, white numbers embossed on a small black plastic rectangle, affixed above the frame with two small metal screws. I knocked.

The door opened, flooding me with the sweet smell of pipe tobacco and the piercing sound of a soprano whose character was probably dying, singing in an opera I did not recognize. Then I saw his face—the smile that made me understand the renewing properties of a smile as if for the first time—and I felt myself become hotly illuminated. I suppressed the urge to smirk, so resounding, intoxicating, and frankly silly were the violins playing in accompaniment to the scene created by my imagination. But as I stood in that open doorway, I felt as though I could see more and more clearly into myself, that I could see my own heart beating and my stomach churning, as though an entirely new internal universe had been opened to me, as if the body's contents might be capable of making sense.

As I studied myself intently in the light of this man's gaze—I hoped he was also awakening to the transformation that was occurring between us—I touched with my mind's hands for the first time those parts of my own body that previously had been absolutely off limits, outside the map of my known emotional world. My cock, my armpits, my anus, my nipples all responded by telling me that I was falling deeply in love—but how could it be?—and that I was finally at the threshold of the journey that I had known I would someday have to make, to that one terrifying place where all was unknown but was mine to be owned. I seemed at last to be filling up the space I had long only partially occupied in the world, which was the first step before moving forward, my now erect cock and nipples heralding the process of my belonging physically in the world. His face beckoned to me to come out, coaxed me to come closer, to stand nearer to him, so I could feel his warmth. "I'm Jorge Arroyo," he said.

I was intensely aware of the smallest movements of his lips and his tongue from the very first moment that he spoke, and I relished the delicate movement of my own organs of voice as I responded. Speech itself was a part of this corporeal transformation, and I felt language penetrating and flowing from me in what before had been prohibited ways, and I flexed the muscles that I used to receive and to produce it. It was as though he were speaking to me through rough kisses pressed passionately to my neck, or to my chest. I wanted his breath in my own mouth, rippling across my own vocal cords, arising as if from my own lungs, helping me to say the simplest words that for so long I had let go unspoken. I wanted syllables to have taste, the flavor of another person's mouth. I wanted to recite all the poems I had never memorized, but which had somehow lodged themselves in my heart. The actual words we exchanged, constituting the inconsequential babble of our shy self-introductions to one another, sadly have become faded in my memory, like old photographs handled too much or exposed to too much joyful sunlight. He invited me in, and as I passed through the portal into his world, it hit me suddenly: this impossibly beautiful face, this gorgeous voice, this *man* was the same one my father had goaded me into meeting, whom I had sworn to avoid at all costs.

When I entered his room, the irony was magnified in the comforting familiarity of what greeted me. My uncanny sense of having been there before went far beyond my recognition of the simple layout and dimensions of the room, which did turn out to be exactly the same as my own; the hand-me-down furniture, the science texts on the desk, the posters, the music all seemed to belong to the home of my own mind and its sensibilities. Instead of my usual reaction to a new interior space, which had always been automatically to heighten my vigilance, to fortify my mistrust, and to fear entrapment—always the paranoid refugee, I had learned well that no settlement could ever seem per-manent, and certainly not safe, to me—I found myself allowing the searchlight of my heart to stop combing the surroundings, and I shut off the alarms of my red ears. The room embraced me physically, a wispy palm in the win-dow touching me with the long fingers of its shadow upon my arm, and the smoke from the pipe in the ashtray brush-ing my cheek as I sat down in the armchair beside it. Our lifelong conversation quietly began.

Tempered by skeletal November, perhaps with the earli-est terrifying reports of a mysterious "gay cancer" swirling around us like the first snowfall at the start of what would be a long winter, we became only devoted friends, at first. The next semester we registered for almost all the same premed classes—he too wanted to become a doctor, which was both greatly reassuring (since physicians by definition could not be queer) and even more intensely attractive (I had always wanted to marry a doctor)—and we became lab partners, thereby establishing the most antiseptic and cere-bral of intimacies. We were suddenly inseparable, forsaking our other friends, which incurred their wrath; in the case of my roommates, their increasingly hostile fag jokes were now plainly directed at me. When Jorge would stop by to retrieve me before dinner, they would send us off with com-ments like "He's all lubed up and ready to go!" I pretended I was too involved in my friendship with Jorge to care what they said, sniffing that our bond was too highly evolved to be comprehended by the likes of them. Yet their bigotry now had the power to shame me, because what they were implying was so likely to be true. Only weeks before, I had been in their enviable position as (ostensibly) white, straight, and male at Amherst, and now, even at the beginning of an exciting new friendship, I felt isolated and adrift. My first response was to seek some limit to, some control over, my budding relationship with Jorge.

Thus our sexual energies were channeled into a kind of competition not so different from what engaged many of our male friends: a game of sorts that was played out on the weekends in the houses and dormitories of Smith and Mount Holyoke. The objective was to pick up the most attractive woman one could find by the end of the evening. Jorge and I worked as a team, charming and wooing and promising return calls, hoping to get invited upstairs. Probably because ultimately we were innocuous and unavailable—the women who befriended us were more insightful than we were, and perhaps sensed we were sexually conflicted—more often than not the end of the evening found us hiding out in a dorm room plastered with glossy posters of hunks. We reliably made the last cut, while my unruly roommates seldom even got through the party's front door. While restoring to me some of my injured machismo, and also forestalling the development of a physical relationship between Jorge and me, these misadventures also sometimes resulted in hurt feelings on the part of the women, whom we had no intention of ever calling back. Though I hardly understood it then, I tried to sleep with these women mostly to impress Jorge, always keeping him at a depth of one body away, fantasizing all the while about what he might be doing in the next room. We also competed in the cutthroat arena of our pre-medical course work. Science was the perfect barrier to self-knowledge, in that it concerned itself only with strictly objective evidence. The laws we studied were not subject to interpretation; each combination of reagents yielded its products through predictable reactions that appeared in stark black and white in our textbooks. Even biology, by comparison with other disciplines the almost disorderly science of life, had little tolerance for deviation from the norm: most mutations were lethal in the unforgiving grand scheme of natural selection. An A in a science course was a measure not simply of one's ability to conform to rules, to isolate the purest product, or to capture the rarest specimen and explain it, however; it also placed one on the path to a successful career not open to the average person. To be at the top of the food chain implied a level of dedication and stamina that only the most genetically well engineered could muster. We laughed at the inquisitive English majors and impressionable art historians who would test the waters in the lowest-level courses, which we superciliously dubbed "Physics for Poets" and "Chem for Fems." They would be the ones frantically looking for jobs after graduation, eventually teaching in high schools if they were lucky, while the best of us would be marching onward to medical school and the promise of large incomes and societal respect.

Gradually, however, in conversation after late-night conversation, chain-smoking together across a small oak table in his room, when the cold was too bone chilling for us to travel to Northampton or even to make an after-hours return to the science complex across campus, we began to peel off the many insulating layers of heavy over-coats and repressive teachers and woolly sweaters and reli-gious guilt and long johns, arguing about what the Greeks meant by their different words for "love" or whether Emily Dickinson was a lesbian, whether homosexuality had a genetic basis or was instead the result of environmental factors. We were considering an approach to what now seems to have been the inevitable next step, rationalizing the need for our nakedness to one another in the scientif-ic terms that were available to us.

We were in many ways willing to educate ourselves despite our assumed callousness, to invent what seemed nowhere to be written down. I began to write poems more hopefully (albeit secretly and sporadically) and resisted the familiar impulse to throw them out immediately. In our pre-medical courses like Chem 12 and Math 21, symbols, proofs, and equations grew paradoxically more and more confusing in their rigid attempts to define the limits of the known universe. While we read as widely as we could man-age outside of our introductory course requirements, still we found precious little to illuminate the elliptical trajecto-ry upon which we had been launched. Even in a required interdisciplinary course called, boldly, "Race and Sex," taught by a Marxist Indian woman whom my parents would have seen as the fulfillment of their worst nightmare, where racial and ethnic stereotypes and traditional gender roles were examined and critiqued, and where I was for the first time not embarrassed to type my real name—*Rafael Campo*, not the bearish, always obliging Ralph—on my research papers, little mention was made of homosexuality.

Sadly, we did not know enough about who we were from our own experiences even to know that we might call ourselves "gay." The few words we might apply routinely to ourselves, "faggot," "homo," and "queer," were like the few words I occasionally borrowed from Spanish: they felt lost and foreign in my mouth and did not even begin to describe what I hoped might make my life more comprehensible. Internally, we only guessed at the depth of expression available to us in the lost language of our hearts, a language that we knew painfully must exist, but for which we had no teachers. At the time, there was no visible gay and lesbian student group on campus, nor even sympathetic articles in the *Amherst Student*. Nor were there very many clues to our existence in the media at large, with the possible exception of the deeply buried, ever more frightening articles on what had become "gay-related immune deficiency" that appeared at shortening intervals in the *New York Times*. It was a new disease that seemed to defy all the rules of nature we were so attentively studying; it struck only those, by implication, who broke nature's laws themselves.

So busily, all the more intently, I graphed limaçons and cardioids in my notebooks for math class; I read with growing intellectual detachment Auden, Bishop, and Merrill for the occasional English class I still felt compelled to take;

and I calculated with precision the energy necessary to turn steam into ice, using thermodynamic principles in chemistry lab. We cultivated as vigorously as we could our identities as premeds—the one thing Jorge and I could be together that was accepted and normal, the one appellation we could safely share. Though I had actively forged a friendship with Jorge Arroyo, a connection that from the beginning I had felt in the deepest recesses of my body, I focused the friendship on memorizing organic chemistry synthetic reactions with him, avoiding the possibility of our own physical synthesis, and always grateful for the tremendous weight of our textbooks.

After the thaw that spring, haltingly, even as we submerged ourselves in our course work, we began to devise strategies to make Amherst a bit more hospitable to us. We made plans to live together during our sophomore year; our flirtation with the idea of rushing different frats was ended, thankfully, when they were all abolished by the college administration. When we then settled on the Spanish House—generally viewed as "queer" because some of the artsier students lived there—we resourcefully justified our choice on the basis of the prime quality of the digs. Thus our first home together was on an island, figuratively at least, separated from its surroundings by a treacherous ocean of cultural differences. Even though we wanted desperately on some deep level to ensconce ourselves securely within the trappings of our own shared ethnic heritage, as the most direct path to intimacy with one another was blocked, publicly we joked about how we planned to divert the money the Department of Romance Languages provided for its nerdy *tertulias* to raging keg parties instead. We would be "Latinos" who listened to Led Zeppelin and not salsa, who preferred pizza to paella, who would be doctors someday and not drug dealers, and who spoke English more naturally than Spanish.

We also planned our seemingly long-overdue summer vacation. To my delight, Jorge invited me on a month-long sailing trip through the Virgin Islands his family was organizing. They had charted a route similar to the one they had taken many times before during Jorge's childhood in Puerto Rico. The tropical geography depicted in the brochures he showed me, with its lush mountains rising dramatically behind long stretches of white sand beach delineating a turquoise sea, promised to allow us to see beyond the confines of our chaste friendship as it had evolved at Amherst. The voyage would also plunge us into Jorge's past, one which had transpired on an island not too distant from the one lost to me, and I imagined the view from the sailboat affording me a glimpse of what might have been my own world. Where else could we possibly belong to each other physically, except perhaps in the throbbing heart of the place where we originated? That mythical place I believed I could never visit, where my father had killed sharks and herded cattle, where my grandmother had prayed when hurricanes ran their hands roughly under her dress, where Spanish was spoken boastfully and freely, where the indomitable sun beat dark colors into the skin of all people. Could such a paradise truly exist?

Suddenly, the academic year ended and we were there, almost naked before one another in our bathing suits, diving into water that was the temperature of our bodies. Jorge's was overgrown with thick black curly hair, almost as densely as the mountainsides were covered in jungle. To my great surprise, he spoke Spanish fluently with his father, as if there were nothing to be ashamed of in a language so musical. Sometimes it was just the two of us sailing at a leisurely pace of our own determination, Jorge shirtless and competently working all the sails and ropes while I lounged on the deck, hardly steering at all, smoking a cigarette. On discovering a secluded inlet, we would sail in part of the way and then anchor. When the heavy weight hit and then caught somewhere at the bottom of the ocean floor, which we could almost see through the deep clear water, it felt like a silent commitment we were making to one another. We stripped, finally naked, and swam off the side of the boat, with not another soul visible for miles, the strong currents in the warm water pulling across our bodies like massaging hands. Amherst College, with its belligerent boozed-up jocks and its drafty wood-paneled classrooms, seemed too distant and unpleasant a memory even to recall, never mind to ponder. Vaguely, I began to dread having to return to the place, which I hardly believed I once would have done anything to attend.

At the moments we thought that we might never go back, or that there was no other place on earth where we had ever existed as a pair, Jorge's father provided us all the reminder we needed. Like my own father, he had grown

impassioned in his admiration of Amherst, both for its conservative reputation and its academic excellence. He was
also an immigrant, but from Argentina, a country whose
tradition of fascism was even more repulsive to me than
what I had been taught to feel for Cuba's communism. So
extreme was he in his devotion to Amherst, he became a
personification of the college on our vacation, asking us
about what classes we planned to take, whom we were dat-
ing, where we would be living. A physician himself, he was
especially intent on knowing our progress in our premedical course work, and though he warned us about the terrible changes that were ruining the once great medical
profession—AIDS chief among them, a disease homosexuals brought on themselves, a disease that was God's judgment on their "lifestyle"—he still held up the profession
like a shining coat of armor that gleamed in the sun, impenetrable, as hard as he was. He treated me kindly enough,
but from the first moment I met him I felt under suspicion
for an unspecified crime. I certainly felt unworthy to be a
friend of his son—especially since I knew nothing about
sailing, spoke Spanish awkwardly, and helped the women
with the dishes after meals. My only redeeming quality
seemed to be that I was helping Jorge excel in his science
courses. Jorge tried to reassure me, saying that his father
never approved of his friends, but I wondered whether his
antipathy toward me reflected what he might have recognized even then as the "special" nature of our closeness.

Though Jorge and I slept together in the same narrow
cabin at the head of the boat—the two bunks met in the

shape of a great V, so that our faces rested only a few inches apart when we lay down to sleep—the snoring presences (especially Jorge's father's) on other levels inside the bowels of the vessel prevented us from going that small distance further. I would lie awake, listening to the insomniac ocean lap against the side of the boat trying to tell me a secret I was on the verge of understanding. It rocked us ever so slightly, almost coaxing us to come together. At those moments, or when just the two of us were swimming or sunbathing together, I felt an uninterrupted connection with the natural world, in spite of Jorge's suspicious father, in spite of what I had been tirelessly taught about homosexual desire's being "unnatural." The sun, the ocean, the sea gulls all accepted us without hesitation, without regard for our attraction to one another. Indeed, the absence of human organization and rules of conduct seemed to give us permission to explore what our bodies told us, even to encourage us to do so.

Everywhere we seemed to see, as if exposed, the warm contents of our bodies. A ripe guava, when opened, revealed our sweet pink flesh. The sky was like vast lungs, the sudden squalls as angry and tearful as I was when we argued about the future. The ocean was our blood, our tears, our saliva, our urine—it mixed freely with all of these fluids as they were produced by us. Our minds were concentrated in the sun, impossible to behold directly, but also burning into our skin what we knew. Our skeletons were strewn across the beaches, the smallest bones were fragments of shells, the long bones sunken into the sand at crisscrossing angles like those of the palm trees. Our voices were modulated but prevailed through the strong wind along with the caws of the brightly colored birds we glimpsed; we seemed physically to have complete expression in this unspoiled, natural world.

When we returned to Amherst in the fall, we brought back with us some of the sun's strength in the golden color of our skin. We had fallen into the habit of speaking Spanish to one another, and we were now in the Spanish House, where other languages were permissible. Our two suitemates—one an African American man whose irreverent manner and peculiar popularity with some of the white frat boys ignited our own suspicions regarding his sexuality, the other a gentle white man from somewhere in Texas whose girlfriend played rugby and was almost twice his size—also seemed to be giving us permission to explore our own unconventional relationship.

Now when we got drunk at Smith or Mount Holyoke, we returned together to our own dorm at Amherst, determined to get there before the disinhibiting effects of the alcohol wore off. Always it was too late by the time we let ourselves nervously into our suite. The weeks flew by, and suddenly it was almost November again. Finally, on Homecoming Weekend, with the entire college worked to a fever pitch over the big football game to be played against arch-rival Williams the next morning, we got so drunk at a blaring frat party that we allowed ourselves to try. While carousing visiting alumni shouted and shattered beer bottles outside our windows, we stripped furtively to our underwear and climbed into my bed. My heart pounded so loudly I thought it too was capable of shattering glass. We lay beside one another, in abject terror, afraid even to touch one another. Nothing happened. About an hour later, Jorge was throwing up in the bathroom, and when he returned to his own bedroom for the night, I was relieved.

The next few weeks provided us plenty of excuses for not talking about what had not happened. Our tans faded. Final exams were upon us, and I was getting killed in my grades—from straight A's in high school, to two A-'s and two B+'s in my first semester at Amherst, and declining into mostly straight B's, with a C even threatening to appear on my transcript for the first time in my life. At times, I was so depressed I was unable to study. Then I would binge on Diet Cokes and Marlboros, pulling all-nighters in order to get a paper in on time. I became increasingly isolated; unable to talk to Jorge, I had almost no one to talk to. I fantasized about suicide as the only way out of humiliating my parents—I was now undeniably a homosexual, my grades were becoming so poor they would prevent me from getting into medical school, and I hated Amherst. They were spending their hard-earned savings on someone who was doomed to unhappiness, a son whom they would remember in the future only as a terrible waste of potential. I was fulfilling all their prophecies for homosexuals, and I had not even had homosexual sex. I was unsuccessful even in the expression of my own hideous vice.

My emotional nadir at Amherst seemed to be marked by a chilling incident that hardly created a wave in the college community at large. One of my peers, known for his right-wing politics, his intellectual arrogance, and a sports column he wrote for the *Amherst Student*, happened to be in an anthropology course on linguistics that Jorge and I were also taking with Mary Catherine Bateson, the famous daughter of the anthropologist Margaret Mead. One day, in a lecture hall containing about one hundred students, during an exercise for which we had to offer examples of certain language constructions whose particulars now escape me, he supplied the following line: "The sick faggot died of the disease." Most of the class laughed uproariously. A few of us cringed, staring into our notebooks numbly, practicing our habit of silence; AIDS had finally made it into the consciousness of college students, even if only to serve as the basis for vicious jokes. Our brave professor, to her credit, interrupted the class immediately. She was enraged, and canceled the remaining classes for the week, imploring us to think about what had been said and our reaction to it, and to examine our consciences closely. When she left Amherst the next year, explaining that she could no longer teach in such a hateful atmosphere, I was crushed. It was the beginning of what promised to be another long winter.

So the few outspoken allies we had were driven off campus; "we" remained an unknown number of gay and lesbian students, invisible except at those painful moments when we were made the objects of bigotry, still without an organization or a voice. Then something unbelievably fabulous occurred, an event of great proportions—fairy-like, radiant, prescient, and reedy-voiced Eve Sedgwick alighted upon Amherst (or at least I was awakened somehow to her luscious presence). She had been hired with full tenure, the rumor had it, almost unheard of at a college famous for denying its junior faculty tenure whenever the opportunity arose. Instantly, she was making her presence known in the Department of English, her insistently sexy ideas like plump hands gliding between the thighs of the grumpy old hard-liners who sat across the table from her in faculty meetings. In addition to the ground-breaking courses she would be offering, with delectable titles such as "Gender and Power in Victorian Fiction" and "Communities of Men, Communities of Women," she would be giving a poetry-writing workshop.

Inexplicably, viscerally, I knew what I had to do. Enrolling in the workshop was like putting on a slinky, strapless cocktail dress—I was preparing to feel desirable again, ready to cross over from the dark world where I felt sealed behind a wall of Amherst's red bricks, to a glorious, lushly vegetated but un–Virgin island perhaps, where I would be available to others in ways that had been impossible for me in the past. Poetry, which I, along with my premed peers, had frequently disparaged, was as forgiving to me as the tropics had been. I beheld its grandeur as if I were encountering it for the first time. Here were rules I could understand, because I could bend them to accommodate my nonstandard dimensions, because they came, finally, from within me, from the same singing interior space where I felt love for Jorge and my parents, where I

felt rage toward my ex-roommates, where I felt a need to
heal that was distinct from my relentless pursuit of admission to medical school. I realized I could make something
of poetry, and not be made by it into something else, as I
often wished science would do with me.

Terrified and overjoyed, I went to the first class meeting
with a sheaf of poems stuffed into one of the pockets of my
oversized overcoat, surprised at how much I had written, and
that it had somehow survived, my heart pounding as forcefully as it had the night I had lain down beside Jorge. I
entered through the main doors of the Merrill Science
Building—the poet's family name had never, until this
moment, been mighty enough to subvert the science I had
always come here to study so diligently in the past. Though
the door that received me was in the front of the building, it
was recessed in a deep black groove in the building's façade
located where its two wings intersected at a right angle and
connected, and now gave me the impression that I was push-
ing in through the *back* door. My perspective was changing,
but on the level of actual physiology and not mere consciousness; those neural processes, which had always merely
buzzed away under the intent glare of the expensive laboratory equipment as I labored, now coursed through me in a
way that was arousing, flowing outward into the world, then
back again to penetrate the innermost lead-lined walls of my
heart so that I could see what it contained.

Hearing our poems read aloud by Professor Sedgwick at
the head of the class like a great white angel heralding our
arrival into our own worlds and bodies, I felt their rhythms

so deeply I was overcome by the feeling that for a long
time I had been drowning. Ever so gradually, like rising to
the unbearably bright surface of the Caribbean after a particularly long dive, so I rose to the surface of language,
urgently, shimmering, naked. I had seen new and unspeakably beautiful things and felt the acute need to describe
them in detail to Jorge, to the whole world. I was out of
breath, yet breathing hard, rhythmically, as deeply as was
necessary to restore this pure oxygen to my tissues, and to
my brain. Professor Sedgwick resuscitated me like a crack
CPR instructor, thumping on my dummy chest, placing
her lips to mine and helping to breathe me back to life. I
was reborn that afternoon, and when I stood up to leave
the classroom my knees wobbled like a newborn lamb's,
and the black linoleum beneath my feet seemed as thick
and tenacious as the black mud of a fertile, rain-drenched
field. I resolved that I would no longer allow myself to die.

   Within a few weeks it was February, and the thaw was
already well under way. Some said it was unnatural, but the
true lovers on campus greeted the change in weather with
joyful hearts. Students walked to class in T-shirts and
shorts, with the snow melting around them so quickly that
it seemed the earth too was impatient to shed its winter
garb. The water rushed recklessly to the storm drains, and
the tinkling sound of a thousand secret waterfalls was all
around us. It was possible now for me to hear music in such
banal things; I was under the influence of Eve Sedgwick,
whose instruction, as any of her students will report, is the
most potent of all aphrodisiacs. I wrote poetry feverishly,

beginning at the outside of my body, running my hands through the layers of tweeds and wool, overcoats and scarves, then stripping them off. By the time Valentine's Day was nearly arrived, my plan had come to me in the form of a sonnet. It was a holiday I had always secretly resented: it provided such hearty and obvious self-congratulations to those for whom, it seemed, love came so easily that it could be prepackaged, while in the flimsy Hallmark expression of my love to my latest girlfriend I had always seen magnified my emptiness of true feeling. This year, however, I knew it would be different.

So on Valentine's Day, on my way to Valentine Hall ("the Chow-line of Love," as it had been dubbed long ago by some of my fellow Amherst men, who pretended to help themselves to "tuna," as they derisively referred to the unattractive women they would facetiously hit on while waiting in line to be served their meals), I hopped across a torrent of snow melt and entered the building. But instead of trying to squirm past the tables set up in the hallways where the baseball team was fulfilling the Amherst tradition of selling red and white carnations—red for someone you loved (or had fucked), white for a "friend"—I waited peacefully in line. The flowers were delivered with personalized messages, and Jorge and I had always sent white ones to all our female friends with cute little greetings that probably disappointed them. The number of red carnations a person accumulated was a kind of status symbol, and I noticed some people carrying bunches of the flowers to dinner. One particularly beautiful woman grinned coyly as she held ten red scentless carnations up to her nose, giggling as she talked to her circle of friends.

When I got to the front of the line, I was greeted by one of the baseball players who looked me over suspiciously. Without hesitation, I placed my order: a red carnation, for Jorge Arroyo. His stubbly face became noticeably paler, and without looking up, he asked whether I was sure I wanted a red carnation, and not white. Red, I insisted. He slid a small white card on the table toward me, reluctantly it seemed, and upon it I wrote a poem and signed it *With All My Love, from Your Secret Admirer.* He quickly pushed the card into its corresponding small white envelope, sealed it, and charged me one dollar. I paid him, and as I turned to walk away, I heard him mumble "Fucking faggot" under his breath.

When Jorge received his carnation later that evening, I was not thinking any longer about the baseball bats that my dollar was going to support, or the specific one that someone might someday wield as a weapon against a queer like me in a dark alley outside a gay bar. I had stood up and made the first public expression of an integral part of my identity, an act that the challenges of my Amherst education ironically made possible. All that I had learned was contained neatly on a small square card, in fourteen lines that sang with my heart and rhymed with my sobs. I had made my honest declaration of love, and so I was oceans away from all the world's dark alleys, I was sailing to the Caribbean in the longer epic I was only beginning to write, the endless love poem that has been my life with Jorge. We met at Amherst College, a small, selective, and conservative liberal arts college in western Massachusetts. Old Amherst, brave Amherst, how can I ever repay you? It was you who taught me how to love when love is not possible, which is also how to heal: now I am kissing Jorge ten years later, as passionately as I finally did for the first time that late winter's night, as we crushed a red carnation between our chests.

A Case of
Mistaken Identities:
The Human Body ⁓

The first thing I learned was how to grunt—I'd like to learn how to float.
    —Seamus Heaney, to a group of young poets

Since art was informed by something beyond its power, all we could enact
was a dance of doubt.
    —Derek Walcott

Duermo en mi cama de roca
Mi sueño dulce y profundo:
Roza una abeja en mi boca
Y crece en mi cuerpo el mundo.
    —José Martí, from "Versos Sencillos"

I remember it clearly, because I heard it while we were trying very hard to cut something out. The surgeon's arms were almost shoulder deep within the abdominal cavity, and he seemed to struggle against being swallowed up by the gaping incision in the patient. His forehead was lightly beaded with perspiration. My grasp on the retractors kept slipping, because my latex gloves were covered with a thin film of blood. They had ordered me to feel the spleen and the liver. As I stood on the verge of slipping into blackness myself—I had heard many stories of medical students fainting in the OR—I found myself desperately attaching myself to a simple sound. I had not even been aware of how intently I was listening to it, and how it seemed to be the only level ground upon which I could stand, until the moment I tried to identify its source. It comforted me wordlessly, and it seemed to buoy me up. It seemed to have been going on forever. It steadied my balance, defining the outline of my tired back like a perfect hand cupped along the length of my spine. Finally, I looked up from the abyss of the sterile field, feeling my neck muscles flex, my eyes reaching toward what was saving me: it was the rhythmic sound of the respirator. In a small, protective glass chamber misted with condensation, its fragile black balloon collapsed and refilled, inhaled and exhaled, made its fist and opened to its blossom, over and over again.

My parents, my premedical advisers, my colleagues in medicine, and even some of my poet friends all have wondered why I am compelled to write poetry, and especially why I bother with so-called formal poetry. They want a clear answer, as much as I do. I have been trying to answer this question for as long as I can remember. It is the surgery I have been performing on myself since I began writing poems, as if I too required assisted breathing the way the patient undergoing an operation to remove a malignant tumor requires the temporary artificial imposition of the innate breathing rhythms. I hear this question as an echo of the external world's ongoing question of me. It is the same question that appears explicitly on every application and every test, college and medical school and residency

applications, SATs and National Boards and tests of standard written English. It is the same question implicitly
asked whenever I pass an attractive man in the street on
my way to work, or when the professor addresses my
pathophysiology class in flawless English. "Identify yourself," this question always demands, "who are you?"

I began by trying to look inwardly at my own internal
organs to articulate my answer, but my spleen is no different in its contours from any other human spleen, and my
brain is just about as convoluted and primitive looking as
the next person's. (I know because I peered timidly
beneath several others' craniums in anatomy class.) Some
of my bones, I have surmised, might be just a little weak-
er, because a trivial skiing accident in high school shattered my left humerus. But it is not until I explore the incision that I am—I sometimes feel myself being cut into
the world when I walk into the wind—or step away from
the gurney to examine my exterior features, that I discover the soft places where this question so easily pierces me.

I have green eyes that seem unusually light against the
contrast of my darker complexion; I had many girlfriends
before I fell in love with a man. My closet contains blood-
spotted surgeon's scrubs shouting their gruff orders and the
collegiate cardigans that deliberate over literature; one
desk drawer is full of fragments of poems I have written,
and another holds the snake of a stethoscope that listens
inscrutably to their rhythms and cadences. I see these con-
tradictions every day in the huge mirror of the world, but
especially on the clearest days, and I cannot escape seeing

myself. I know I once stared blankly at my own body in the wood-framed mirror on my bedroom's blank wall when I was a teenager, trying to figure out which parts I wanted, and which others differentiated me from other people and thus should be amputated. Except I did not know how to amputate then.

I mostly grew up in an affluent New Jersey suburb. I was the darkest note in the white harmony of classroom after antiseptic classroom—I worried that I made discordant sounds when I smiled or played. So I listened very carefully, to whatever was humming and throbbing in the environ-ment at all times, as a way of validating my existence. Maybe this is more simply called heightened alertness, or perhaps even paranoia. I marveled at what I heard; I became fascinated, even obsessed by sounds. But I often wonder whether what I hearkened to was an echo of Spanish mur-muring rhythmically in my head, an incessant but inaccurate replaying of those horrible (yet oddly comforting) albums my father sometimes played, filling the evenings up to the stars with warm hands. The merengue singer's laments seemed directed at me personally, their exaggerated sadness related somehow to my distance from them, their plaintive voices' energy and inflections becoming the fleshy arms that could pull me almost gravitationally back to Cuba—the only place, it seemed, that I could never, never visit.

I was continually embarrassed by who I might be then, as if my classmates had invisible ears pressed to my family life, so that they might hear that same Spanish blaring from the crack under my door. I remember the fluorescent lights in the eerie classrooms I once shared with mostly fair-skinned kids, the long sleek tubes of light laid together in the shallow, upside-down graves of the ceiling. I felt backwards and exposed in their brightness, as they buzzed all the time their commentary, telling me not to sing aloud, because it was the United States of America all around me, urging me to repeat the Pledge of Allegiance, which I had memorized dutifully. My classmates seemed to be saying secret things to one another in each morning's solemn monotone: "I pledge allegiance to the flag. Don't be proud or pompous. Don't be different. Don't be musical. Don't be a sissy. Don't speak Spanish." Just like their muted, cool voices, the strange lights seemed the condensation of the absence of a tropical landscape, a sort of eternal snow raining down, burying me in a harsh winter light.

As a sad child I learned voraciously, eating up knowledge to fend off the starvation of my spirit. I knew I was "different," and in more ways than anyone could discern, so I learned my new language very well. I began telling unbelievable stories and writing poems early in life, and I wonder whether my obsessive impulse to write was even at its earliest manifestation a rebellious one, engendered by an unconscious desire to revise the world according to a discordant internal reality I was trying so desperately to decipher. My cardboard report cards, like my bed and all windows and every classroom, were each another in a series of squares that contained me. My parents rewarded me generously for all the A's that were neatly held, like me, in tiny square boxes, and I pretended to be happy.

My favorite sport in those days was soccer (it seemed to me vaguely important that this was a popular sport in Latin America). I marveled at how American kids seemed to like it. It was a game with straightforward rules, yet I could make something with it from the movement of my own body. I played the game passably well, and I fixed my mind, while running on the autumnal continent of playing field with the trees wildly on fire all around me, on getting by my powerful kick the beautiful arc right so that the bouncing patchwork soccer ball would enter the rectangle of the goal to the applause of the crowd. When the frenetic ball would finally rest, tangled and seeming terribly deflated in the thousands of small boxes that made up the net, it was a tremendous relief to see a thing of such savage motion become so utterly trapped.

In a similar sense, in spite of myself I have always wanted to enter the dependable squares of New England. I wanted to fit the way the square peg fit into the board of the very earliest of my preschool toys. Even now, I can still stare myself into the pattern of the red bricks in the buildings of Amherst College when I return there as an alumnus. I like to stand in the middle of the main quadrangle, and from this vast square look out over the well-groomed playing fields to the panoramic pulsations of mountains, where the language of the land is expressed all along the horizon. The words of great poets—Dickinson, Frost, and Merrill—I suspect have always been physically present everywhere in these surroundings. For four years they exerted their iambic pull on my heart, conversing directly with my internal organs, most of that time without my even knowing it.

Long before I understood what college was, when I was still a small child, my family moved to Venezuela rather unexpectedly, with the news of my father's transfer to manage a subsidiary company owned by the larger corporation for which he worked. "A good opportunity for you to learn Spanish," he said, or threatened. I was terrified by the prospect of traveling to a place that might more closely resemble a home, where I could unpack and breathe more definitively, where I would play with huge spiders and crack open coconuts. Even though we lived there for only a short period, the move precipitated violent headaches in me, which I recall vividly—they were the atomic explosions of all that light and the new environment into my head, the heat and the gigantic sun, my subterranean language of Spanish now suddenly spoken loudly everywhere, the unpredictability of all things, even the shapes of leaves. The crazy playgrounds where iguanas unexpectedly dropped from the trees and the sky! There were unforeseen, horrible metaphors and invisible creatures in the very sounds of the exotic language I suddenly dared to speak aloud. The words seemed to touch each other in forbidden ways, in the same ways I was discovering I wanted to touch and be touched. I was only nine or ten at the time, so with these headaches I may have been demanding attention—or pleading to be returned to the flat, rectangular pavement of the playgrounds in America that had begun to give form to my imagination.

Though I do not remember feeling uprooted or home-sick, I know I was quietly afraid—afraid, perhaps, to be set free in a place where I was expected to know the way, but where I feared not having the right directions. I was afraid of my own true home, afraid of what I was discovering I so intensely desired. I was afraid my stomach might swell up, even explode, like the distended bellies of the malnour-ished children I saw running naked in the streets of Caracas, who in other ways resembled me more than did the friends I left behind in suburban New Jersey. Despite intensive medical and psychological study—including the oddly reassuring experience of having my brain imaged by a machine whose walls enclosed me in a space not more than six inches beyond my nose—the experts my parents consulted never found anything wrong with me. The last of the mysterious and unbearable headaches struck on my final airplane ride back to the United States, and I have never suffered from them since.

When we finally returned to New Jersey after several years, I hoped that nothing much had really changed in me except that I had glimpsed a real jungle; if I was in any way different, perhaps I had merely swallowed too much South American dirt, or been unknowingly stung by a poi-sonous insect. In time, I was able to compare what I had seen to my own internal version of the jungle, that dark tangle of slithering intestines and organs heavy as overripe fruit I hated to admit were inside me. I began to perceive more consciously that my task in growing up, like that of other persons born into an unfamiliar environment that

they by necessity must call home, was to transpose somehow the internal onto the external, to wed my chaos with
the orderliness of those around me.

I thought that I needed to create a safe nest that would
bear me in its heart through the long, white winters, where
I could have the brick walls on which I had come to
depend, but which could be lined with cozy bits and
shreds of my native flora. My most private, innermost bed
could take the shape of that exuberantly unpredictable leaf
that I saw beckoning in Venezuela; I also brought back the
obscenities of Spanish words, but continued to speak them
only in my head. I reassembled them with the ceaselessly
modulating, echoing container of my English voice box,
feeling how I used my mouth and my stroking tongue, the
most sensual organs in my body. So began my fantasy of
describing in a novel language of my own creation the
secure habitat in whose hidden bat-filled caverns and tow-
ering treetops I would dwell from that moment on.

Whereas I had been called Ralph all through grammar
and high school, I suddenly was transformed into Rafael in
college. Whereas I had been cleanshaven, I let grow a
bushy mustache my mother once remarked made me "look
like a Mexican." And as for the flamboyant orchid of my
sexuality—I had been attracted to men for as long as I
could remember—I stopped plucking it before it could
open to all of its magnificent colors. Now when I breathed
in the Northern Hemisphere's frozen air, I saw that what I
exhaled might be hot smoke. I was on the brink of a great
discovery; I was young Columbus traveling backward

through time, not into the unknown but toward a place I knew too well yet had somehow forgotten. Even so, even if I sensed I was more liberated in my nascent self-awareness, I realized just as acutely that by figuring out how my heart worked I might be all the more capable of self-destruction.

Poetry thus at first became a way of *deliberately* applying boundaries and barbed wire to these "new" aspects of myself. I wrote terrible poems, choked by frequent caesuras and off-rhymes and precipitously enjambed line breaks, my carefully worded stanzas stacked just as carefully as a kindergartner's wooden blocks, but still I congratulated myself that at least I was writing, at least I had found a place to start. At the same time, I prepared myself for my career in medicine—the largest, most rigid box of all those I had encountered and could help to construct—in another effort to comprehend, and perhaps to contain, my blossoming. Perhaps the glowing image of the CAT scanner, and the way it had once investigated me so effortlessly and painlessly, its invisible fingers combing through my murky interior, attracted me. And if either of the paths of writing or medicine could lead to the respect and admiration of others, then that was even better. The idea that people might come to have of me was comforting in its flatness, in its perpetual two dimensions, in the thin, depthless volume of verse or the frame of the simple word "Doctor" preceding my name.

Writing workshops became the ears to the chest through which I could hear more clearly the sounds poems were making; medical school would soon allow me to ultrasound the human body. The two, I pretended as I filled in the blanks on my medical school applications, were really connected. I tried to fashion a single school of high-walled Gothic architecture in my imagination, an uninterrupted hallowed hallway through which I could pass in one directed process of learning. Surprised that I was even admitted—a neuroscience major who declared a major in English as well, a scientist whose lab experiments failed but who also wrote a thesis of original verse—I proceeded to enroll in medical school, full of the youthful arrogance my parents labeled idealism. With the semiconscious purpose of helping to heal medically indigent populations in this country—the shadows of the taut-bellied Venezuelan children will never leave me—my mission would be to prevent the ailing human body from failing to keep time.

I know I wrote my first deliberate poem to my mother because I wanted her to stop crying, so she could breathe more easily, the way I must somehow remember she did when she carried me hopefully inside her body. In the lifetime from fetus to physician, these unsophisticated impulses—to express and to live—still seem closely related to me. Both poetry and medicine, when properly and honestly practiced, are attempts to reintroduce that familiar sense of order into an environment gone out of control—for me, at least, they are the same effort to create a figure of my design, for once, upon painful experience.

What grew inside me throughout medical school, however, was a strange and unsatisfying relationship to language I did not expect. The healthy impulse to look inside was for a time corrupted by insiderliness. I began to wonder whether the stirrings I felt inside myself might not be the viable fetus of my desires given flesh at all, but rather represented some unborn potential in me doomed always to lurk, defying expression and impossible to articulate, an unintelligible language to which I would never give voice with the rhythmic contractions of birth. There it was, the horrible monster of my early poetry, the only thing I could possibly parent, the frightening product of some misguided experiment where the sperm of a poet fertilized the egg of a scientist: yet I yearned to feed my awful hybrid muse, and resolved always to keep it chained up very close to me.

So, once I arrived at Harvard Medical School, I quickly reinventoried my needs. I desperately wanted to learn the inner language of the human body, and to have the kind of fluency that comes from tracing the surface of the liver, in the way the Venezuelan heat that hummed with the Spanish language seemed to dramatize living, making obvious the burning metabolism within my own body. I wanted to learn how to mend my broken arm myself, to make from words a skeleton to give shape to the body of my experience—I wanted to make a cast to protect myself, to straighten myself out again, to keep me correctly aligned. I wanted to hear the rhythms of breathing deafeningly amplified by my stethoscope. I wanted to pick apart the vocal cords through a laryngoscope and examine the anatomy of the eardrum and the tiny, protruding ossicles through an otoscope. I wanted to descend even closer, even smaller, and step down the tunnel of a microscope to hear the ions ebbing and flowing across cell membranes, and the incessant beating of cilia. I wanted, in short, a scientific explanation for the mystery of the voice—a distorted, pathological corollary to wanting to use my own. More and more, I wanted my own voice to be defined by objective and material constraints.

But by the end of three long years of medical school, I had never seen a reason to write poetry through the microscope. Cuba seemed just as incurably distant as ever, and the naked body grew all the more elusive. Science, my hero and my one sure thing, seemed to be failing me. The equations I memorized began taking up the space of poems I had learned by heart in college. The sheer amount of data I was expected to assimilate was staggering, and I was being flattened—again, but in a different way since now I was actively, even gleefully cooperating. Some of the horror stories I had heard about medical school were beginning to come true. I was becoming the very monster of my own poetry, one who killed bloodlessly, silently, with the most surgical of wounds; I was becoming what in my most frightened moments I had always dreamed of becoming, another instrument of precise algorithms, a sharp metal tool by which the exact distance from health to disease could be calculated to within three decimal places.

The more I feared that medical school was not providing the supports I needed to reimagine myself more positively, the more I avoided the very mechanisms set in place by the medical school to assist students; I got only so far as the waiting room of the University Health Services counselor's office, where stale *New Yorker* magazines seemed to have been deliberately strewn about to remind me of my utter failure as a poet. I was consciously and explicitly forbidding myself the application of heartfelt, *meaningful* language, even internal dialogue, to what I was doing. I was withholding words in the same way that I commanded my patients to hold their breath, I was carving and shaping language into artificial lines and stanzas in a scarier version of the cosmetic surgery I had studied and seen performed. Control became the medium in which I was entrapped—I was like a sculptor entering his stone, but never returning with what he's found. My beautiful Gothic architecture, with its resounding hallowed halls and its whimsical gargoyles, was becoming a garish disguise for a silent, very bleak prison.

My writing itself became transformed, and like a medical student who begins to diagnose in himself the diseases he is studying, so too did the few poems I managed to write become more and more diseased. What had begun as an attempt to define began to defile instead. Most of the rhyming mnemonics I employed to learn the pathognomonic signs of illness were vulgar and distasteful. I began to conceal the fact that I wrote poems at all, because for the first time it seemed not simply a private activity but a subterfuge, a devious and subversive threat to my medical career goals unless I kept it in line. Poetry soon became my dirtiest secret, and I feared being exposed as a poet more than I ever did seeing "send back the wetbacks" or "faggots die" spray-painted on the brick walls around Harvard Square. (Even now as I write, I still shudder slightly at the thought of "coming out"—as an artist.) After the first two years, I finally stopped writing altogether. I concentrated all my energies on saving what was left of the container I still needed medical school to be for me. I worked harder than ever and, paralleling the pattern of my early childhood, did well enough in my rotations.

It was my surgery rotation that jolted me away from my path toward relentless self-enclosure. Ironically, at first it must have been the labyrinth of the surgical floor that so attracted me to surgery—its rooms within rooms filled with tiles, the gray locker room brimming with locked compartments, literally to the ceiling. The surgical floor, its automatically closing doors always sealing tightly behind me, transmitted the message that "everything is under wraps"— even microorganisms were screened out of the ORs by the infinitesimal meshwork of their air filters. The strong hierarchy of the surgical team also appealed to me intensely, and I convinced myself that their casual homophobic and racist jokes were funny and the abuse was well deserved— after all, I knew too well that I had a sentient body and thus desperately needed to be controlled.

Then came the day in the OR when I discovered myself clinging to the respirator as if it were my own heartbeat and I had never been born. By the end of that lengthy operation, I felt as though the huge tumor had finally been cut out of *me*. I looked at it, entranced: a bloody, contorted mass lying in a perfectly sterile, square, mirror-like metal pan. At that moment, I did not know what was worse, to live recklessly as the tumor did, exceeding its own walls and almost killing the patient who carried it, or to have brutally excised it the way the surgeons had, placing it like a prize framed in a cold specimen dish to confirm that it was now incapable of hurting anyone.

What I saw was an excised tumor in a sterile specimen dish. My staring began to transform it, until I saw the shape of an impoverished island bloodied by revolution in a dazzling sea. Then I saw the castrated penis of an accused homosexual cast upon the cold stone floor of the Inquisitor's jail. Finally, I saw not a thing at all but the seething, healing word itself, the crucial chapter of a human narrative that would change a life forever. Then, with the same suddenness and blustery effort of the cured patient as he came up coughing from the depths of anesthesia, I understood what I needed to do.

I needed to accept that I have always been hopelessly in love with the muscularity of formal verse, the way it can wring meaning from the patchwork cloth of my life, one that I still fear might wear itself out from scrubbing the messy floors of a society desperate for homogeneity. Writing good iambic pentameter feels like putting stitches into the anonymous, eternally gaping wound of being human, and rhymes can be intertwined like surgical knots. To write formal poetry is sometimes even a way to sew myself into the body of traditions from which I sometimes feel excluded, as if I were an amputated clubfoot yearning to have its blood supply restored. If I can make English rhyme and sing, if I can be graceful and seamless, maybe I can touch the gleaming shell that rests on the beach of my Cuban heritage, the conch that when blown has always seemed to me to produce sounds sung in the melody of Spanish. If I can write a decent sonnet, maybe I can bring my hand to my lover's chest and stroke it with the same passion an English gentleman might have felt as he passed his warm hands across his lover's heaving breasts.

I am startled often by the moments when I glimpse my imagination pedaling along in its rhythms like the child I once was on my bicycle; I am amazed when I observe these rhythms actually corresponding to the tempo of the exterior world. I dream that these rhythms are all fundamentally the same. I want to become immersed in these rhythms and to strike only harmonious chords. I want my language to echo those rhythms, I want my sexuality to be a normal variation, I want to be a good son and a good American. I want to be my own hero, the armored Spanish sailor who never sank and drowned with the Armada but washed up miraculously upon England's shore, and at the same time the red-bearded Celt who gave my father's Spanish grandparents their blue eyes—I know these historical people are all versions of the one history I want to reincarnate. I want to hear myself think clearly, and I want my parents to listen. I want to be heard, to stand on the stage at the center of human attention, where all the drums are beating. I desperately want everyone in the world to understand the Spanish I almost never learned, and I want to master English myself, indisputably. I want to write in the entirely new language of my own country, the United States of America. Perhaps paying the utmost attention to rhythm, meter, and rhyme can make these deep childish wishes come true.

I have adult reasons too for why I continue to be drawn in the direction of formal poetry. It too is a complex science, with its own elegant arguments, a practical system with rules I can trust. I can try to measure my experience with it; I can use it to plot graphs of my emotions, so that I can hold them up later to study more carefully, and I can use it to harness the energy of the furiously pounding heart. With it I may make connections across centuries and across identities to other artists, as when I quote Wordsworth and Traherne and Herbert. I imagine I can be taken more seriously in the world of poetry, since in the discerning eyes of his medical peers a physician who writes poems is certainly suspect—soft, impossible to prove statistically, not rigorous enough in his proofs.

In a parallel universe, medical science may also be a way of controlling and understanding the physical processes of the human body, a way to wrap my hands around life—my own particular, peculiar life feeling so unanchored at times. Yet here is where I have learned that the hazard lies, where the powerful fusion can blind. I once thought, wrongly, I could calculate race in terms of melanin; I guessed I could measure sexuality by cross-sectioning the hypothalamus. In laying my hands upon the ethereal bodies of hypothetical patients, I even hoped I could touch my own body. I supposed if I could purge their bodies of infestations with antibiotics, I could be a whole, unitary, and cleansed person myself. In curing them, I half believed, I could ultimately cure my own maladies. If medicine is indeed a kind of poetry, it is a poetry endangered by hubris, with its too many answers and explanations and footnotes and analyses, which need to be tempered with the awful reality of blood and the actual stench of urine.

Now I realize that for a long time what I had feared was my own humanity. The sound of my own voice had frightened me, as if I had been walking down the dark alleyway of my trachea alone at night; by humming and whistling to myself I only imitated life, instead of creating it, when I first tried to write poems. I had never been in control of my environment at all—I merely created the illusion that I was. I began, not realizing it, *without* the hope of being that peg that fit snugly into the board—I see now that I always was the monstrous, pink-mouthed iguana lurking in the closet, I am the truth that I was always afraid to tell. The most affluent suburb in America could not change that. Years of hygienic classrooms could not change that, nor could peering out into the razor sunlight from half-shut doors and windows. Even "returning" to Venezuela to discover my heritage was a long-winded lie, told by an airplane that transported me so close to, without ever actually reaching, the sun. My schizophrenias are what I am, the active process itself. There is no medication to cure me, and only boxes of my own construction to contain me, whose walls allowed me to smash against them my own head.

That day in the OR I decided to try to answer the question of why I must write, putting all the facile answers of
history, and genealogy, and careerism aside. As I sat in the
stillness of that yawning, tiled cavern of a room, listening
with awe to my own regular and thoughtless breathing, I
knew that the very act of living itself was the source of
energy to write poems. Music and language were suddenly my sweet internal instruments, not enslavers to be
appeased, nor the empty promises of an escapist, unearth-
ly identity. I could scream in my voice like hands all over
their golden words and grammatical rules, in the same way
I had once dreamed of touching them. Spanish and
English were immediately the same, they had the same
sounds, they were spoken in the same mouth, and they
lived in confluent gyri on my temporal lobe. Being gay was
joyfully not to have a country of origin at all, only a place
in my heart where a man was extending his arms toward
me. I could take possession of each sound in my own
mouth, and be lifted up to a new hilltop that was in no particular country, but one I could nonetheless visit and
demonstrate to the world. I did not need medical school to
show me that my eyes see into the world by their own
physiology, or that my own neurons encode and transmit
my experience; I have been seeing and seeing all along.

I can see that I am something new and that from me I
can extend my naked arm. The form of the bone, which
healed long ago, gives it a peculiar shape. I no longer want
to amputate it, or to rebreak it and set it in a better cast.
Now I give myself the parts of me I never understood and

never liked. As a poet, my challenge is to create myself, in my own image, using the corporeal materials common to all speakers of English; as a physician, my challenge is to accept the absolute necessity of that process. Words are indistinguishable from my physical body now. I hope to fulfill a similar role for my patients: I want their words to come forth as if from my own lungs. I want to hand them back, as I examine them and talk with them, their own bodies with their distinct, troubling features attended to, cared for, studied, celebrated, and discussed. Sometimes they will be cured—a spine set straight, an abscess drained. Sometimes they will die unexpectedly. But these extremes identify only small corners in the larger drama of healing. In the middle of a single life, and in so many other cases, what I am naming may be their real need: someone to listen only to their breathing, then to their hearts, to hear the universal human sound each one of us, alone and together, creates.

Fifteen Minutes
after Gary Died ~

I want to write about AIDS . . .
I haven't really written about what I look like now.
I have a new skin. I have a new identity . . .
There is a geometry to this, a poetry too . . .
       —Gary Fisher, from Gary in your pocket

He was utterly irresistible, yet something kept me at an arm's length. It was a warm day in San Francisco, but at a table full of bared forearms and elbows, freckles and golden tans casually brandished over baskets of warm crusty bread in the pool of sunlight the restaurant's windows afforded us, he had his shirtsleeves rolled down over his black skin and buttoned carefully at his wrists. I remember thinking his wrists rather delicate, finely made. The occasion was Eve Sedgwick's forty-second birthday— her message on my answering machine several weeks before had been enticing, even more enticing than the high-pitched sound of her breathy voice always was: "I want you to meet my dear friend Gary. He was a graduate student of mine at Berkeley, right after I met you. He's the most talented writer I know. He'll be coming to the party."

Having been thus disabused of the richly enabling fantasy that *I* might be the most talented writer Eve knew, I petulantly resolved to go to her little fiesta to meet this little Gary person. I prepared myself to be very unimpressed, even a bit petty and mean-spirited, though I admitted to a few of my friends that I was curious to meet him. I rehearsed a few spiteful one-liners: "Oh, so you're a writer. Didn't I see something of yours in that obscure regional publication called the *Orphic Lute?*" Maybe she meant fiction writer and not poet, I thought in an attempt to repair my slightly damaged ego, or whatever was left of it after nine months of internship. "So you write short stories. How do you know when they're short enough?" I was quite prepared.

The days before that gloriously sun-drenched table was gathered had flashed by, as I was up to my ears in my usual patient care responsibilities. I worked with a machine-like indefatigability. I was finding myself to be more compulsively driven than was usual for me, partly because of totally unfounded rumors circulated by some of my peers that I was among those under serious consideration for the position of chief resident. Rather than feel insulted if they were only jesting—such cruelty was to be expected among a group so starved for appreciation—I allowed myself to half believe them. To be selected for this position was one of the very few accolades given to medical residents, and I felt myself being easily seduced by the possibility. I had especially admired one of the chiefs during my internship year. She always placed an emphasis on humane and compassionate care for patients first, without compromising decision making based on an extensive knowledge of cutting-edge medical theory, and at the same time teaching both actively and by the sheer power of her example. I was trying to model myself on her; she was one of the minority of physicians around me who demonstrated that these qualities were not necessarily mutually exclusive. Many of the others seemed more intent upon comparing the length of the lists of their differential diagnoses than on knowing anything about who their patients were outside of the hospital.

I had come to the University of California at San Francisco from Harvard Medical School in large part because the rich palette of the patient population—Asians, whites, Latinos, openly gay and lesbian people, and African Americans, and within each of these groups, even further layerings of ethnicities, nationalities, and political views—exerted a powerfully attractive force upon me, on a conceptual level. More important, the city struck me as a truly progressive place where differences mattered in a positive way and where constructive dialogue took the place of shrill name-calling. My partner of eight years had already obtained a position in the ophthalmology residency, and he was irrepressibly thrilled at the prospect of our living together in San Francisco. So I gladly left the stately brick buildings and frigid streets of Boston (where in the newspaper I had once seen photographs taken in Southie of signs reading "God hates fags" wielded as weapons at the first Saint Patrick's Day parade in over a hundred years that had permitted openly gay Irish American participants to march) to the painted-lady Victorians' pastels and rainbow-flag bedecked streets of San Francisco, where I imagined same-sex couples strolled holding hands and smiling, requiring no special holiday, or court injunction against the city, to do so.

Gary, I found out as we slurped oysters from their iridescent shells, was far more advanced in his appreciation of San Francisco's fabled diversity than I would ever be— apparently he'd slept with men of nearly every race and creed, including one particularly conflicted Muslim man with a huge cock who suggested before they went to bed that Gary put on a veil, which he later used to tie Gary up. I was aghast, but titillated and transfixed; I greedily slurped two more oysters. Needless to say, my stupid *Orphic Lute* comment had gone virtually unheeded, rolling off Gary's brilliant exterior like semen on a mirror, which was the salient detail from the next scandalous story he was already busy relating. Gary went on about his romantic escapades, ending with a long lament about the white men in his home state of North Carolina, who were still hung up on all the history in that master-slave thing, making it entirely too boring to enjoy. I must have appeared entirely overstimulated, perhaps quivering a bit, oyster-like, surrounded by what had grown to be a large pile of emptied shells, because across the table I noticed Eve beaming in my direction, which she was in the habit of doing whenever she had a hand in overstimulating anyone. I recognized that satisfied look from her writing workshop.

Gary did write short stories, it turned out—*and* poems. In fact, he spent the rest of our time together essentially spinning outlandish versions of them for me as we shopped later that afternoon for CDs—we both gravitated independently to the International Music section, which he said was proof of our essential compatibility. He introduced me to Zap Mama, an Afro-European a cappella group, which he said I should listen to before it appeared on Arsenio's or some other tired old queen's talk show, thus to be deemed "hip." Later I tried unsuccessfully to find a rare Two Nice Girls CD, but this was Tower Records in the Castro, so of course they were sold out. He looked at me dubiously, anyway, knitting his brows over what he probably regarded as the hopelessness of a gay Latino man listening to what he interpreted from my description to be a bunch of boring white lesbians from Tennessee singing about love and commitment. "They sound worse than the Indigo Girls—but at least they're out," he groaned.

It was Gary's own completely natural and unforced "outness" that so captivated me at first. I had never seen anything like it. I watched with envy as he shamelessly flirted with the cute punked-out green-haired guy at the register, coyly complimenting him on his nose ring. He wanted the eyes of the world on his body, on his smile, on the spectacle of his easy, angelic interpenetration with other people's souls. He spoke with absolute confidence about his writing, as if there were no question but that I would be interested in it. And of course I was. Even though his most obsessive themes were potentially divisive and explosive—from what I could gather during our conversation, they ranged from the interplay of race and sexuality to the relationship between creativity and power—he spoke with such animated enthusiasm about them that they took on the universal appeal in my enthralled imagination of the most accessible of fairy tales. Most of all, his creative work seemed acutely relevant and absolutely necessary, in contrast to the impotence and futility I had come to attribute to my own pitiful attempts to marry writing with doctoring. Gary was all of his conflicting, ebullient, sexy, and angry identities, effortlessly and at once—and, in spite of myself, I was falling for each and every one of them.

We parted then, before the oddly romantic antitheft device at the exit of the store, scribbling down our addresses and phone numbers for each other on scraps of paper. At some point during the afternoon, we had promised to send each other some samples of our writing without ever actually saying the words. Gary, of course, had a P.O. box where he said he had all "the juicy stuff" sent. I was overcome by a sense of inadequacy, never having had a P.O. box myself, having always been too reticent to read the personals, pornography offers, and phone sex ads in the gay papers even while I glanced furtively over the seductive pictures that accompanied them. I was still afraid at that point even to subscribe to gay periodicals, fearing some list kept by the government, which conceivably could communicate with the American Medical Association or the Department of Medicine at UCSF. Together and absolutely committed to each other from the beginning of our sexual lives, our wider social life suppressed by such fears and the demands of our medical training, my partner and I had become an inviolable (and hopelessly square) gay "community" unto ourselves. Though I was elated to be in a place where gay people were more visible, I hardly knew personally any other gay men at all.

As Gary swept down the stairs leading out onto the street, turning his head with eyes widened by exaggerated delight as he tracked for a few moments the progress in the opposite direction of a striking, lightly made-up drag queen perhaps out on a few afternoon shopping errands, I was struck by a sense of the tremendous amount of space he was taking with him. Then he spryly turned the corner and in the next moment was out of my sight. I contemplated what I had gained and so suddenly lost. Somehow, the whole afternoon had felt shadowy and illicit, which made me feel strangely empowered in spite of myself and all my well-practiced inhibitions. The world was sparkling and new again, and I felt like a teenager living inside the diamond of as yet unmade discoveries. I had met Gary Fisher.

Perhaps it was my giddiness that had prevented me from noticing at first. In any case, soon I was mercilessly plunged back into the depths of my medical training. The next two months were particularly grueling, as I saw more and more of my patients die, most of them of AIDS and its complications. Later that summer, when my resident at the other end of the telephone line at 2 A.M. announced I had another "fag fever" waiting for me in the emergency room requiring admission to the hospital, I hardly noticed the anger and frustration in his voice, because on some level I shared it. I slammed down the receiver and skulked my way down to the ER, where behind a thin yellow curtain an African American man lay outstretched on a gurney. He spoke not a single word to me. For the several hours it took me to complete his evaluation and admission paperwork— I took my time, as some kind of twisted imaginary revenge I could exact upon this stubbornly mute obstacle to my sleep—I was nagged by a feeling that I knew him from somewhere. Much as I wanted to see him as just another uncountable, indistinguishable AIDS case, arms marbled with KS lesions, wheezing and sputtering as he tried to inhale a hissing nebulizer treatment, no-not-anyone-like-me-or-anyone-I-knew—suddenly, and with a kind of brutality that seemed not blunted but magnified by my exasperation, it dawned on me. I thought of Gary, a glance I had at the restaurant of the same type of blue corrugated respiratory tubing, snaking its way out of his satchel. This man reminded me of Gary.

Indeed, I had not given a thought to Gary in many, many weeks. My initial infatuation with him had been met immediately with my fail-safe mechanisms for repression. I had neatly and efficiently converted his campiness into effeminacy, his raucous humor into poor taste, and his sex-

ual confidence into a self-destructive addiction to promiscuous sex. His smile created special problems for me,
because it seemed so inexhaustible and was so immediately endearing, but with much work I had made it somehow
seem sinister and predatory. I had loathed myself intensely (as soon as the glow of that early intimacy had faded)
for considering even for a moment that I might be attracted to him. After all, I was an overworked and therefore
self-righteous physician, and for all intents and purposes
neither gay nor Latino at all, so certainly I could not identify with some trashy black queer who deserved whatever
filthy disease it was that he had contracted, who probably
had—and so it hit me—AIDS.

In fact, I had busied myself with ever greater fervor in
my attempts to impress my colleagues, which had left me
little time for writing and even less for pursuing a friendship with the likes of Gary. Contrary to what San
Francisco's diversity of patients had led me to expect, I was
being taught and had almost already learned to ignore the
role of sticky psychosocial issues like sexual orientation,
race, or ethnicity in medical care—one such effort of mine
already had led to an anonymous hand-scrawled note
placed in my evaluation file saying that I had "problems
with identifying too strongly" with my patients, and "the
tendency to let my emotions get in the way of patient
care." (The attending physician who I presume wrote this
assessment of me had made some disparaging remarks
about a male-to-female Latino transsexual under our super-
vision who eerily happened to share my last name—I had

objected strongly to his comments and attempted to gen-
erate some discussion of homophobia on rounds, noting
that I myself was gay.) I had decided after that sobering
incident to keep my gayness, as well as any other "tenden-
cies" I or anyone else could identify in me, strictly to
myself. I was relearning the correct and appropriate use of
silence; even if AIDS could make gay people as a group
more visible in some ways, it could also drive us more
deeply into hiding.

So I pored over my cumbersome medical textbooks
instead of reading poetry, and I went to interns' and later
residents' report with interesting cases—and if they were
AIDS cases, with the plan to discuss only the exotic para-
site or reportable bacteria and never the humanistic
dimensions that frequently also complicated the illness—
prepared to present to the gray-haired attending physicians who called me Raul or Ramon instead of Rafael, if
they even noticed me. I know that on some level I had
already lost a great deal of confidence in myself along the
way, every "fag fever" and mispronunciation of my name
taking its small but measurable toll, but by the time I finished internship and started residency I thought I might
still have a chance of being recognized, of standing out.
When I received the news that my manuscript of poems
had been selected for publication in the National Poetry
Series, a manuscript I had submitted with a sense of des-
peration before I had even graduated from medical school,
instead of crying out with elation, I cringed, wondering
how negatively this would impact on my medical career. It

seemed an undeniable confirmation that I was queer after all—creative writing not only was a distraction from hard-core medicine but was itself soft, too empathic and frighteningly loving. The ethic under which I toiled was that anyone who had time to write about his feelings certainly was not spending enough time searching the medical literature for relevant articles and memorizing the data.

The next time I really saw Gary he was all the more larger-than-life, but under the terrible magnifying glass of an ICU. It was in a hospital outside of the UCSF system. Now his arms were unceremoniously bared, left uncovered by the flimsy hospital gown, revealing the extensive patches of the all-too familiar KS lesions; now a blue corrugated tube in plain view connected him to a ventilator. His once delicate wrists were swollen and bruised, and I surmised that some distraught intern had encountered great difficulties in finding veins for his IVs. A calendar with black numbers so huge they became grotesque hung on the wall across from his bed, marking days he lived through but would never remember. It disturbed me, how much I was being forced to see. In the ICU rooms I had been in before, the groans and gurgles had not come from a body with a face I recognized; nor even, it seemed, from a suffering person: they were merely the sounds one heard at such proximity to death.

Eve's telephone call the night before had indeed been ominous, and her voice on my answering machine this time subdued and almost vacant: Gary was in the hospital, could I call her at the Hilton in San Francisco, she would be arriving that night, Gary had AIDS. My denial remained profound, even as I studied the monitor that displayed his vital signs, a reflexive action that suddenly became an intimacy almost too great for me to bear. Not because of any fondness I harbored for Gary, which I had nearly succeeded in extirpating over the previous several months, but because now for the first time I actually and personally knew someone with AIDS. In my selfish experience of that moment at his bedside, I felt the shock as though I myself had received the terminal diagnosis. No longer could I consider myself immune, or invisible; it was as if my own body's defenses were suddenly as pulverized as Gary's, and my own decrepit body lay outstretched before me.

I took some solace in the fact that I was sure, after seeing him connected to so many blinking and beeping machines, that he would quickly die; at least I would be saved the trouble of actually having to get to know him better. One law of medicine I had learned well during my tortured internship was that the number of machines surrounding a patient was inversely proportional to the chance of survival. I cagily read over his chart, displaying my medical ID prominently on my jacket almost as a shield, going so far as to lay my stethoscope out on the desk where I read (though I had no intention of examining him), lest anyone mistake whose side I was on. His nurse only scowled at me, probably thinking I would end up creating more work for him. Gary had been previously hospitalized, I was dismayed to learn, several times at a smaller community hospital in Oakland to receive chemotherapy for KS so widespread it was thought to involve his lungs; he'd also had pneumocystis pneumonia twice before we'd even met at Eve's birthday party.

Slowly, bits of my sketchy history of knowing Gary resurfaced. The buttoned-down shirtsleeves and blue tubing returned more vividly, along with the musical cough brought out by his laugh, the telltale prominence of his cheekbones. The feeling I had that he had a serious question to ask me—in fact, hadn't Eve mentioned something to that effect? The holding back of something, made more palpable by his natural openness and warmth in our conversation during that brief afternoon shopping spree. The imploring look he gave Eve as they said good-bye, which gave way to an impish smile, the smile I had remembered and so expertly reworked. How I had turned my face to the side to avoid kissing him on the lips when we parted outside the music store. Suddenly, I was acutely aware of Gary's enforced silence over all those months, a silence I had conspired with him to maintain.

The next night I returned to the ICU, where I found Eve at Gary's bedside, distressed but at the same time appearing as solidly in control as a pilot in her dark closed cockpit of dials and digital readouts. I coaxed her out of Gary's isolation room and then proceeded to explain to her what I thought Gary's chances of surviving were. I spoke as bluntly as I could, a seasoned soldier sparing none of his war-weary pessimism. I suppose I was wishing Gary away, desperate to have the whole mess come to a closure and

thus to avoid ever having to deal with AIDS humanely,
more than I was answering her questions. I made a great
point of inquiring whether Gary had been "made DNR"
yet—Do Not Resuscitate orders are written in the medical
chart after discussions with family and friends, or with
patients themselves, indicate they do not wish aggressive
therapy in the event of a potentially terminal event—and
I felt once again the brute power over patients implicit in
that medicalese expression. Surely Gary would not want
his life to be prolonged in the condition he was in at that
moment, I supposed aloud, though the little I did know
Gary led me to believe that the opposite was probably
true, that he was probably a fighter. Eve said very little,
though I craved the sound of her voice making its way
across these decisions.

The next day I did hear her voice, bright as the sunlight
I found when I walked into Gary's new room, which had
miraculous windows with a sparkling view of downtown—
he had been transferred to the regular medical ward.
Earlier that morning, the ICU team had extubated him
successfully, to almost everyone's surprise. Except Gary's,
of course—he sat up in bed presiding over the chaotic
scene, a bit groggy, but commanding his sisters to confess
to him how much they loved him. And so I was introduced
to Leslie and Luchina, as beautiful physically as Gary, nearly the same proportions of male and female characteristics
but expressed through women's bodies. Immediately, as I
had when I first met Gary, I found myself falling for them,
my defenses melting away in the bubbling potion of their

speech. They seemed tired, and I almost could calculate how long Gary must have been sick, the entire course of his illness visible in their drawn faces. Still, they were cheerful, welcoming me warmly into the circle of their experience, generous with everything except their pain. Gary, perhaps sensing how taken I was with them, piped up: "Oh, it's that gay Mexican doctor."

So I found myself on the other side again, but this time not so much by my own choosing or complicity. How eager I was to avail myself of *these* aspects of the human experience of AIDS, the closeness and warmth of an embattled and grateful family, the joy at the miracle of survival, the persistence of a familiar voice! But it would not be so easy for me. Gary had deliberately not spoken my name; maybe he had forgotten it. He also challenged me by placing alongside one another two identities I had been laboring to keep separate, and throwing in an approximation of a third. He did not even deign to apply the label of writer to me, an omission I felt acutely. He had managed in a single remark—and post-extubation, no less—to humble me more than any of my stupidly rehearsed one-liners had affected him at that distant lunch party where we had first met. I managed to make him see, through my cloud of guilt and repression, a thin smile.

"Rafael," I said. "We met at Eve's party, and you were supposed to send me some of your stories." Before we could say anything more, he fell asleep.

Gary floated in and out of consciousness that day, the effect of which was to endow him with a decidedly ghostlike ability to hear what was being said about him without the speaker's knowledge and then comment on it much later. He was haunting his own hospital room, he said, joking that he had almost died, so he was entitled to do that—he qualified for a special discount near-death learner's haunting permit. So when Leslie, Luchina, or Eve would tell a story about him, full of particulars like charmed amulets to ward away death, an hour or two later he would interrupt an unrelated conversation to revise a certain small detail, saying he had been caught wearing his mother's and not his grandmother's negligee when his father came home early that night, or that he wrote that short story not in Berkeley but back in North Carolina.

Later that week, when we did talk in more depth—he continued to improve dramatically with the chemotherapy he was receiving for the KS that had progressively involved his lungs and that seemed to have become particularly aggressive during his course of therapy for a superimposed third case of pneumocystis pneumonia—he likened that state to his process of writing. Eavesdropping on the world around him without anyone's knowing it, then recording what he had heard and seen—that, he said, was what he did when he wrote. It gave a certain illicit, irresistible quality to his writing. And he was continuing to do it. Upon his bedside table were stacked several thickly bulging "journals," and competing with them for space were the small leftover bowls of ageless Jell-O cubes and half-drunk glasses of cranberry juice, which I always handled carefully, as I was still unaccustomed to not wearing

latex gloves around AIDS patients. He filled these notebooks with everything, from sometimes unflattering
sketches of his visitors to letters finally written after years
of pent-up emotions to garish descriptions of the places to
which his illness had brought him. The urgency of it all
was in the tremulous handwriting, in the earthquake language, in the aftershock bloodstains. I thought of him
refusing to put aside his work whenever the tensely thin-
lipped phlebotomists arrived, the blood he was pouring
into his writing clearly more precious than the sample they
would want to draw and then take for analysis to the lab.

My first encounter with Gary's work was reading these
remarkable journals, often while he dozed in his bed just a
few feet away. I was an interloper, a fugitive in his pages;
even though I used as my invitation to read them our distant mutual promise to share our writing with one another, I still felt that I had to read them surreptitiously. The
delicious intimacy of his mouth, my ear being brought
together into such close proximity by those pages—that
was how I learned to stop seeing Gary as a dying man who
needed my pity, for whom I should grieve. His writing sustained in me the mixture of joy and resentment I had experienced on meeting him; he made himself more and more
human to me on the page, ever more contentious and gos-
sipy and irreverent, obsessed with eating and laughing,
shitting and pissing. Nothing of the unattainable, unsul-
lied, and regretful self one usually encounters in eulogies,
particularly those written by the dying person himself.
This work was too busy figuring out how it was alive, how

it was persisting, and by what unfathomable processes the disease was trying to alter that tenacious life. His descriptions of his body's sensations, from swallowing a large pill to expelling a liquid stool, all were struggled with, all fully engaged and experienced. Whenever Gary awakened, he would smile at me, pleased by the extent of my awe. Our jointly policed moratorium on words had finally been lifted, and I for one was overjoyed.

I began to be infected with AIDS myself, I imagined, to need the virus in the same physical way as I came to need Gary's voice. I wallowed in my own fantasized illness with Gary's help, for the first time in months allowing myself to identify not dangerously but joyously with someone who was suffering, and thus thwarting the effect some of my residency evaluators had been having on me. I was completely self-indulgent, cultivating and tending to the KS growing in my lungs and on my skin, feeling the pitter-patter of the tiniest pneumocystis organisms in my airways, the insidious suffocating feeling prompting me to cry out with whatever happiness and pain I discovered in my heart, the new purple blotches on my arms an embodied refusal to remain invisible. I did not feel important at all, I discovered, but rather marginalized; "the sick role," contrary to the assumptions implicit in that awful medical school term, was not a perfomance a person put on at all but a constrained space to which one was assigned, and which one occupied at great expense to one's self-esteem. But there were ways, I was learning, of making it larger.

Imagining AIDS was not just an effort to reeducate

myself; it was also a form of self-punishment, even atonement. I realized through my growing friendship with Gary
and the metamorphosis it effected in me how many facets
my guilt displayed. Not only did I woefully regret the hostility and the destructive impulses I had felt toward my
patients with AIDS—the anger I harbored toward the
epidemic itself having somehow been distorted and
rechanneled through my sleep-deprived psyche toward
those suffering in its wake—I also felt guilty for having
been spared. Since Gary and I had so much in common, it
seemed tragically unfair that he should be so ill, and I
healthy. Our shared passion for writing, our shared experience of living in the shadows thrown upon us by the
darker shades of our skin, our shared struggle with being
queer in communities of color for whom gayness and
AIDS each represented "white diseases"—all of these sim-
ilarities, once so unrecognizable, enabled me too readily to
see myself in Gary's place.

And yet I had not, until now, found the time to get to
know him. The M.D. after my name, so long interposed
between me and the world of the infirm, that professional
appendage sheathed in protective latex, an anti-penis
designed to keep me disengaged, sexless, AIDS-free, and
possibly straight—M.D., the brusque abbreviation of My
Desire, only served to heighten my guilt. Not only was I
improbably aligned with a medical bureaucracy that
denied me; I was also shamefully powerless to cure. Worse,
my prognostications were inaccurate, as was evident by
Gary's very animated, and flirtatious, smile. So I saw that I

lived to no end; I lived only to hear one of my colleagues whisper to another as I walked away from a casual conversation: "Can you believe it?—I heard he was gay. Too bad, he really seems like such a nice guy."

Some of my guilt was even less rational. I felt guilty for my monogamy, thinking myself too self-loathing to have become liberated sexually in the way Gary had set himself free. My devoted and patient partner, the single greatest joy in my life, endured these flagellations somehow. I also felt guilty for not having found the time to do more research in relation to AIDS, though I was working up to eighty hours a week. I felt guilty even about my ongoing efforts in the writing of poetry, which seemed so inadequate a record of the devastation, so obviously self-serving and self-indulgent. My book in progress was a source of unbearable agony, because it felt so much like playing a horribly out-of-tune violin while San Francisco was burning all around me. Each poem was the slightest of whimpers, the rarest clearing of the throat, when what I wanted to bring forth was a voluptuous scream, to vomit in the various shades present in Gary's basin. I compared my own demoralized writing with the poetry that was responding more exuberantly to the epidemic, such as the work of Thom Gunn, Tory Dent, Kenny Fries, Michael Klein, Richard McCann, and Mark Doty, somehow managing to celebrate the life going on despite AIDS. I read Gary's journals, and I wept, and I laughed aloud.

When I left Gary's hospital room that morning, only to return to another hospital in a few hours the next day in my usual role, I had already unconsciously begun to alter my approach to the care of my patients. My thoughts of ending my own life, which had risen as quickly in my mind as had my intense feelings of guilt, were subdued by the challenge I sensed in the work that, I had finally realized, still lay ahead of me. I found myself hoping for some kind of redemption; I searched my patients' eyes for it, I listened for it in their hearts and lungs, I pondered the possibility of it as I interpreted the scans of their brains. Gradually, over the following weeks, the two hospitals no longer seemed such vastly different worlds to me; the person I was, entering each one day in and day out, was evolving from a split personality into an integrated whole. To witness Gary growing stronger over those weeks, responding to the chemotherapy enough to be sassing the nurses who administered it, was to be cured myself.

Gary went home after a few more relatively uneventful weeks—a permanent IV catheter was placed through his chest, and he rode out several high fevers for which no source was ever found. (Gary joked that even with the awful, limp catheter in, he could still be very hot.) His sisters and his friends arranged everything so that he could receive chemotherapy, antibiotics, nursing care, even meals at home. Whenever Eve could fly into town, the two of us would visit a whole evening with him, all three of us lounging in bed together like teenagers at a slumber party. Gary wore a brightly colored cap over his stubbly scalp, though his hair had already begun to grow back. He also wore a blue turquoise necklace that Eve and I both coveted; each round stone appeared to be a slightly different miniature version of the globe. But only Gary could wear entire worlds as jewelry. We passed a camera around, shooting photographs of each other, which soon turned into mostly shooting photos of Gary. The camera adored his face as much as we did. The experience of taking these pictures of him, focusing on his dazzling smile or the dramatic tilt of his head, contrasted starkly with my usual method of imaging people with AIDS, which usually involved radiation and looking inside them for the hidden pathology it was a foregone conclusion that they must contain. Feeling the power of seeing into their brains and lungs, without ever noticing their faces—that had been partly how I had lost sight of my patients.

Though I am somehow still reluctant to admit it—it is extremely threatening for most physicians to be in any way indebted to the sick, since they must always be paying us— Gary became my role model for the care of patients, by the way he cared for himself and those around him. He helped me remove the mask I wore in the hospital and in my clinic, which revealed me to be no less human than my patients after all. I could stand naked beside them, as I asked them to do when I would examine them. Gazing into Gary's eyes, feeling a kind of love that was at once platonic and erotic, pure white light and full of the colors of our skin and our irises, permitted me to look into my patients' eyes without the need for my ophthalmoscope. Gary, even when his sources of energy were so diminished by his struggles with the virus in his blood, still managed to suffuse the pages before him and the people around him with a love that declared itself not to be temporary. It was as irresistible and all-encompassing as the process of dying itself, and yet it was antithetical to death.

I think my friends in medicine sensed some of the changes occurring in me. Whatever dedication I had to the care of patients, particularly people with AIDS, was multiplied in my rediscovery of it. The resurgence of my spirits was met by increasing talk about my prospects for becoming chief resident—although now, ironically, such recognition mattered less to me than it had before. If I stayed late in the hospital, it was because my patients needed me, not because it looked good. I read less of the medical literature and more of June Jordan, Paul Monette, Marilyn Hacker, Audre Lourde, and Randy Shilts. And, of course, more and more of Gary Fisher.

Fueled by my new connection with Gary, I made the time to serve on a committee whose aim was to increase the diversity of the house staff, and ultimately the faculty, in the Department of Medicine at UCSF. We gathered in the late evenings to discuss topics ranging from strategies for recruitment to increasing acceptance and tolerance for minority physicians already in the program. The initial discussions were encouraging, although I was soon jarred out of my complacency, when I found precious little support—in a room full of people clearly dedicated to promoting diversity—on the issue of gays and lesbians in medicine. There we sat, in a room with mahogany paneling that was oddly almost the same shade as Gary's skin, for the first few

moments after I had spoken in total silence, when all I had
suggested was that the committee make efforts to identify
and to recruit gay and lesbian people.

In the next instant, I found myself being lectured quite
reasonably on how "homosexuals" were already too powerful in San Francisco, that San Francisco was a magnet for
"gays" already, that gay and lesbian people did not face the
same economic barriers to success and so were not
oppressed in the same way as Latinos and African
Americans, that being openly gay was a choice and so
need not interfere with one's applications to residency programs or one's professional advancement. My experience,
in fact, had been quite the opposite—despite trying to
remain closeted, I had suffered far more degradation at the
hands of homophobes than I had ever borne as a Latino.
But I found it impossible to defend my point; my voice
seemed frozen in my throat, and even thinking of the flu-
idity and persuasiveness of Gary's prose could not liberate
it. Apparently, my opinions were needed only as a Latino
in that room, and not as a gay man.

My feelings about diversity seemed rooted in what was
happening to Gary as much as in what had happened to
me. Gary had never had a black doctor, nor one who he
knew was gay. His journals contained harrowing tales of
being kept waiting endlessly and ignored, and even
harassed and mistreated, by health care workers from nurses to physicians to EMT's. I knew of more than a few
instances of such discrimination—my own shameful and
misguided behavior in the San Francisco General

Hospital's emergency room, my attending on the wards who made nervous jokes about our transsexual patient with AIDS, proposals to segregate privately insured and medically indigent patients on the wards, other house staff whom my friends and I had heard casually toss off racist and homophobic remarks.

So in a residency program where the most common complaint was that we were burdened with having to care for "too many" AIDS patients, who were almost all gay men and people of color, it seemed to me the least that could be done was to ensure that the house staff resemble as closely as possible the people we served. (Ironically, it was "too many" AIDS cases because of the way it skewed the opportunities for learning medicine, and not in sad or angry recognition of the devastation of the epidemic.) I did not believe in the niceties of diversity for the sake of merely filling quotas for groups the government officially declared to be underserved and underrepresented; rather, I believed in creating an atmosphere where all people, patients and physicians alike, were respected because of who they were as people. The only way to accomplish that goal, it seemed to me, was to attract excellent people from a variety of backgrounds in order for us to educate one another.

I knew that "creating diversity" was not a perfect solution to the problem of forging empathy out of so many clashing human identities. I had only to remember my own gradual withdrawal from most of the social aspects of the residency, and how in turn I had failed to educate the mostly well-intentioned people around me. I had my usual excuses—that there were far too few of us who were openly gay and could thus stand up as a group against homophobia, that culturally I was more comfortably upper-middle-class white than Latino or gay at all, that too much of my precious time was already consumed by caring for hordes of the needy and alienated who were supposedly my brethren. Still, I had to believe in a cure for our mutual dis-ease; my friendship with Gary demanded that. In my own self-righteous way, I also believed that I could forgive people for their ignorance and their blind terror, if they in turn could forgive us for being merely who we were.

Forgiveness and the yearning for it were central in Gary's writing, and shaped his struggle to go on living; violence and punishment were key narrative elements in his fiction, the most desperate means to absolution. In his more personal writing, he was never the object of anyone's pity, certainly not his own, nor did he seek pardon for his actions. It was as though he inhabited a separate realm, where justice was automatic and came naturally, like a birthright. His writing implied that dying was the ultimate form of forgiveness, because after it there can be no further blaming, and there are no greater consequences. Medicine, as intent upon assigning guilt as upon making the correct diagnosis, provided Gary with a wealth of opportunities to forgive. He had no choice but to accede to the exigencies of his situation. Among his friends and family—from the abusive father who had disowned him years ago to the ex-lover who had insisted on knowing him ever more deeply and ended their relationship when Gary could reveal no more, to me in my perpetual tardiness and unavailability— Gary wandered, bestowing upon us the possibility for self-knowledge that recounted rather than judged, that understood rather than accused. I felt my richly accreted and elaborated guilt dissolve instantly in his gaze.

His writing gave voice to what I unmistakably heard and recognized as an entire language of forgiveness, in that it made no accusations. Through all the various layers of oppression and frank violence, I kept finding myself understanding why. The voice would sometimes withhold itself, then return in fits and starts; there were many places where he simply stopped speaking, where a poem ended cliff-like in mid-stanza—perhaps he was unable to go on, perhaps he was censoring himself in the way he had been so brutally taught, perhaps it was at those moments he felt his own life being cut short. The opportunities for rage were abundant, and certainly rage and even despair found ample expression in the work, but ultimately it was Gary's utter decency and sweetness that burrowed its way into my own heart. Even when writing about sadomasochistic sex, as he did in one of his best stories (entitled "Arabesque"), even when he helped me to explore the darkest terrain of my own sexual fantasies involving violence and degradation, he did so with inexplicable tenderness, as though attending to a wound. Critical to him in his creative work and in the telling of the narrative of his illness were not the pain and the suffering themselves, but what they could teach us about arousal, love, and compas-

sion. His was a voice of universalization, not marginaliza-
tion—of inclusion, not scapegoating—which seemed
directed against precisely the powerful forces that pro-
claim incessantly "they are getting what they deserve."

Of all the great gifts Gary gave me during the last
months of his life, perhaps the most valuable has been the
forgiveness he gave his own body. He wrote about his
body not in an attempt to understand it but perhaps as a
way to extend himself physically into the world after his
death. He not so gamely took in each medication, drawing
the colorful pills in his notebooks as he downed them,
thereby linking what he wrote as directly as possible with
what was going on inside his body. Each word traversed
the purple patches of KS as it passed from his brain, trans-
mogrified through his arms and fingers onto the page, on
its way to the representation of his experience. His body
betrayed him, and yet was him, infiltrating his writing like
the exuberant and reckless blood vessels overgrowing his
skin. Gary knew better than to attempt to revise himself in
those pages after pages of laments, frustrations, joys,
humiliations, and victories. He wisely allowed himself the
space of one forgiven of everything, for whom there are no
expectations or attendant failures, whose only responsibility is to imagine a world without suffering, and then to suffer. The availability of his suffering brought me as close as
I could ever come to the suffering of my patients, for
which I had always been so quick to blame them; my own
relation to AIDS, I discovered through the generosity of
Gary's spirit, was not as victim or as agent of affliction after

all. I was free to be simply who I was. Guiltless, but with a responsibility of my own to help.

The last few weeks of Gary's life brought this process of recognition directly into the path of my medical career. After several weeks of my absence—I had begun the most harrowing month of my residency to date, on the CRI (also known in residentspeak as "the Cry of Pain," CRI standing as an eponym for Cancer Research Institute)— the messages I received from Gary, Eve, his sisters, and his friends were growing more and more urgent. I knew Gary's condition was deteriorating; I could hear the effort he made to speak in the few breathless sentences that seemed almost unable to hold themselves electromagnetized to the tape in my answering machine. Not that Gary's charisma was waning. He always managed a joke about where I might be, wondering lasciviously whether I might be at work late "servicing" one of my patients, at a special rate higher than what was charged for a regular office visit.

He was not joking about a request that I thought we had put to rest months before: namely, would I consider taking on *his* case, as a consultant of sorts. I was already a veteran of my family's and other friends' frequent soliciting of medical advice, usually about matters of diet, minimized aches and pains, new medications and high-dose vitamin supplements. My response was simply to refer them to their regular doctors, especially if a level of physical intimacy was required that was absolutely too daunting—I categorically refused to examine any part of a family member's body below the neck and above the knees. I suspect-

ed that on some level my aversions reflected my distance
as a physician from people in general, and that perhaps the
idea of a patient who had actually seen *me* naked (however
long ago) was too threatening, but it also seemed to make
good clinical sense that my emotional connections to
them might cloud my judgment.

My difficulties in Gary's case had nothing to do with
any residual physical revulsions at all. By then I could
bring myself to take a sip from his coffee cup, could forget
that I was not wearing the medical world's ubiquitous latex
gloves when I held his hand. Indeed, in his body I saw
many features that belonged possibly to my own, and I
had unabashedly fantasized about an even greater physical
closeness and interchangeableness than what we already
shared. My reluctance to be his doctor had more to do
with other unresolved feelings I had reshelved when I had
started the CRI. The extent of the unmitigated suffering
and dying of the "end stage" cancer patients around me
had in an instant caused me to rally about me my familiar
defenses. Though I spent many hours in my patients'
rooms, trying to find any far-fetched, overwrought, and
remotely rational explanation I could for what was happening to them, I inevitably felt more like their jailer than
like their ally. Most of my time was spent dictating dis-
charge summaries, often in connection with patients who
had died, or would soon die, having "failed" (as was the
medical term) their experimental chemotherapy. The one
teaching session we were to have on issues of death and
dying, to be given by one of the attending physicians

whom I admired most for his recognition of his own and his patients' humanity, was canceled at the last minute as the service was so unexpectedly and uncontrollably busy—providing me, it seemed, only one more opportunity for unguided mourning.

Whatever emotional resources I had hoarded during my reeducation at Gary's hands had been exhausted in my first few days on the CRI. Wanting to appear strong— "strong" being the term of utmost respect that the house staff reserved to describe that most desirable quality of cool competence in a resident—I sealed myself off even from Gary. I saw his persistent calls as an unwanted burden, forgetting those long afternoons reading at his bedside, glimpsing an understanding of myself at the exhortation of his example; on a few occasions, I allowed my answering machine, whose recording of my voice was more cheerful than any live greeting I could muster at the time, to take his calls while I dozed emotionlessly on the couch. I had traveled far away from the now unimaginable scene of my re-creation as a gay Latino physician, that vortex of Gary's writing and experience where medicine was mixed with queerness, blackness with empowerment, and AIDS with undying love. I had returned to the antiseptic, blindingly white hospital, where sex absolutely was not possible or relevant, where shit was an emergency to be cleaned up *stat*, where blood and sweat were counteraggressions and occupational hazards, where death was an unwelcome, unforgiven bastard of a presence to be battled at all cost.

What happened next was impossible to have predicted,

as most dramas in the emergency room usually seem to me in retrospect. As if in an attempt to get my attention, Gary ended up at UCSF, finally unable to breathe at all, after placing a desperate call to 911, where someone always answers the phone. Had he arrived at the hospital just two or three hours later, he would have been my patient, according to the scheme by which new cases are assigned to admitting residents. By the sheer force of his illness, as if it were somehow aware of what Gary wanted, as if Gary even at this late stage of the disease still managed to control and harness a bit of its destructive power, the relationship of doctor to patient was nearly imposed upon me. The screaming sirens of the ambulance more than made up for his lack of breath. Now he would be heard.

He was in the hospital for several days before I even knew he was there. I discovered it only when I overheard the intern on the team taking care of him complaining about having to explain everything in detail to his new patient. This difficult patient also refused to eat the hospital food, and had requested that a sign be posted on his door requesting anyone wishing to enter to knock before doing so. Most disconcerting, however, was how he kept himself up late into the night writing in a thick spiral notebook; surely, the intern surmised, he was recording names and all the information he was given so later he or his family could sue in the event of a bad outcome. My eyes darted over to the board where patients were listed first by room number and then by last name; I was oddly not at all surprised to see Gary's in the box for Room 1105.

It was another day or two before I could identify myself to anyone as a personal friend of Gary's, nor did I find the courage to enter his room to visit him until he had been hospitalized for almost a week. I did, however, avail myself of his chart and read through the record of his admission. His chest X ray done in the ER revealed both lungs almost entirely suffused in fluid, thought to have arisen from the KS, which had found its way back into his lungs, threatening again the very source of his voice. A chest tube had been placed to drain the bloody effusion, and the plan was to blast him with more chemotherapy, since the tumors had responded so dramatically during his previous hospitalization at the outside hospital where I had visited him in the ICU. The tube passing through his chest wall was excruciatingly painful, and Gary was voluble in letting the primary team know about it. He was viewed as a "pain management problem," and guessing by my own resistance in the past to providing pain medications to patients I had presumed were "drug seekers," I wondered if he was being heard. I recalled Gary's saying that not only did most of the clinicians he had encountered assume that as an African American man he had been exposed to AIDS by intravenous drug use, but they were also exceedingly reluctant to treat his pain with adequate doses of narcotics, for fear they were being manipulated into feeding the habit they almost invariably attributed to him.

When I finally crossed the threshold into his room, it was late at night after all his visitors had returned home. I was greeted by the bubbling sound of the pump that continued to suck the fluid from his lungs, and the enchanting sight of Gary in bed bent over his journal, writing by the light of his bedside lamp. The details of our conversation, which was very brief, have been worn down almost to nothing by the flood of my emotions, which has poured over them countless times. He was pissed off. He was in pain. But what I remember most clearly is that Gary forgave me, again, and then sent me back out into the world as an embodiment of what he thought might be possible to change in that world, that alien place AIDS had created for him, and now for me, to decipher. He knew I could not agree to be his doctor; I was still trying to figure out how to be his friend. He forgave me my own needs, understanding at once my preoccupation and fascination with his death and my fear of its consuming me. In that tiny hospital room, on my own turf and surrounded by devices familiar to and workable only by me, fairy-godmotherly Gary orchestrated with the sweep of his pen my salvation. Capable of levitating above his bed, lashed down only by the chest tube that attached him to the mortal world I inhabited, he made me feel fabulously and unabashedly queer, made me want to sing the soothing Spanish lullabies whose words I knew but had never learned.

I visited more frequently during his last week in the hospital, proud of knowing him and telling anyone who would listen about his extraordinary writing. The outpouring of support I felt from my true friends in the residency program, those people who had recognized better than I had who I was from the start of our friendships, softened the blow of the news that came later that very same week, news that Gary's deterioration had somehow foretold—I was not among those selected to be chief resident. So the consolations I received were for two events that I had never had the ability, intelligence, stamina, or foresight to control—the imminent death of a dear friend, and the most petty and mundane of career disappointments. My fantasy of becoming chief resident seemed all the more pathetic and ridiculous in the light spilling across Gary's page, emanating from that bedside lamp.

Now I know I can no longer deny that I have inherited his various struggles. Now I own "all the hurting shards of relation and identity," as Eve herself has put it. I have cut my soft doctor's hands on their razor-sharp edges as I wrote this essay. I was shattered and added myself to those shards at the moment when everything slammed to a halt a few weeks later, after Gary had been discharged from the hospital to home hospice care, when with Zap Mama playing low in the background as I collapsed on my couch after a long day on the wards, my last telephone call to this as yet unknown and incomparable writer reached instead his sob-choked brother-in-law at his bedside, about fifteen minutes late to hear what might have been his last spoken words. I had called to listen too late—about fifteen minutes after Gary died.

AIDS and the
Poetry of Healing ⁓

Now you were tired, and yet not tired enough—
Still hungry for the great world you were losing
Steadily in no season of your choosing—
And when at last the whole death was assured,
Drugs having failed, and when you had endured
Two weeks of an abominable constraint,
You faced it equably, without complaint,
Unwhimpering, but not at peace with it.
You'd lived as if your time was infinite.
                    —Thom Gunn, from "Lament"

The coughing fits continued to worsen until by
three in the morning he was doubled over on himself,
sweating copiously, almost unable to talk. He likened the
pain in his right flank to a hot knife. An invisible torturer
stood beside his bed, silent, red-eyed, and mechanical, as
tall and malevolent perhaps as one of the digital infusion
pumps by which he was receiving intravenous medication.
I rubbed my eyes as I hovered above the bed myself, listening to his lungs, listening to his story of the pain: when
it came on, what made it better, what made it worse, how
much blood in the sputum and for how long. In between

deep gasps for air, he labored to talk about his hometown of New Orleans, and other fantastic places he had been, what in life had made him happy, what had made him sad, the blood he had once seen on the pavement at an ACT UP demonstration. Then he read me a poem a friend of his had written for him, and by the time he was done the coughing ceased for a few moments.

I ordered a chest X ray, trying to feel some of the magical power of being able to see into another person's body. Or maybe the feeling of doing something, anything at all, was what I sought. I could hear him start coughing again in his room across the hallway as I wrote, sitting in a comfortable chair in the doctors' lounge, my assessment in his chart. Hemoptysis, fever, pneumothorax, pulmonary embolism, tuberculosis, pneumocystis, Kaposi's sarcoma. Not a word about his New Orleans, his wry self-description ("I'm as delicate as a hot house flower"), the angry demonstrations he had attended; nothing about his race or sexual orientation or the clot-red roses wilting on the bedside table. No mention of the invisible torturer, either, or why he was dying. In short, no mention of us. The story of this pain belongs to all of us, I realized as one-handedly I snapped shut the chart.

When I was in elementary school, newly returned from living in Venezuela for a few years, a bunch of my new classmates in suburban New Jersey beat me up, calling me "faggot" or "spic," I cannot remember which. That was the first time I saw blood come from my own mouth, red like anger and shame, hot like strangely salty vocal tears. Some

other relevant facts are these: I experimented with drugs in
high school, but I was afraid of the needles. I was experimenting with sex before high school, but I was afraid of
the older boys. I wrote poems secretly, hiding my notebooks in my closet. I thought about killing myself, because
those poems knew that I was gay. I graduated at the top of
my class and went on to Amherst College. I once made
love in New Orleans, in a hotel room beneath a handprint
on the ceiling, to a Puerto Rican man. I planned a career in
medicine, spending a year off doing basic science research
on the AIDS virus. I quit the research job, partly because
it involved killing far too many albino lab rats and "har-
vesting" their eyes, and partly because I could not see the
point of all that pressure to obtain positive results simply
to advance one's reputation or to find another money-
making drug that does not cure AIDS. Eventually I finished medical school, instead of doing graduate work in
English, because I hoped to work directly with AIDS
patients; the epidemic had already taken root. As a third-
year student on the wards, I stuck myself with a needle
during my medicine rotation. When I came down with a
fever and cough two weeks later, I thought for the first
time, and the millionth time, that I might have AIDS
myself. A year later I wrote a poem about the man whose
blood I was drawing at the time, who died of AIDS
because there still is no cure. I went to Roxbury,
Massachusetts, as part of a community health center out-
reach program, my heart pounding as we distributed condoms to teenagers over threats from adult passersby. Last

night, after a chest X ray was taken of my patient from New Orleans—which revealed nothing—he died, before I could tell him any of this, before I could say that in some deeply unspeakable and complicated way I loved him.

I know that, like my patient's symptoms, these bits of my life are related; I want to provide a complete, honest, detailed history, the kind of history I expected from him when he came to the emergency room. Then I want to assemble the information obtained under a single, unifying diagnosis. Except in the end I lack a specific disease, or the name for one. I want to say AIDS, or high-risk group, or empathy, or queer, or Latino, or "it hurts here." I want to say, "Doctor Campo, heal me." I want to take an X ray of myself, and to see not just the bones I will leave behind someday but directly into my ghostly soul. Or write a poem that miraculously cures AIDS in every language, every culture.

Instead, day in and day out I draw more blood, and then write fragments of iambic pentameter that are incomprehensible to me when I return home late from the hospital—though their rhythms alone, at times, might lull me to sleep. Oftentimes I cannot seem to find a decent vein, or the right words, so I stab blindly. More pain in that. The patients insist that it does not hurt, always giving more, always wanting to be understood. And yet I am speechless; my tube is empty. I have nightmares sometimes that I am drowning in blood, that blood is too plentiful, that there is so much blood I can sink a bucket into it, blood flowing like rich red satin sheets rolling in the wind, blood that tastes sweet instead of salty, blood pouring from my mouth like a mournful Spanish song, the blood of my ancestors telling its most precious and guarded secrets, how much potassium, how much sodium, the composition like that of the minerals in Cuba's fertile soil. Sometimes the blood is an angry ocean, and the virus is floating on the surface, visible, like a tiny sailboat, or a child's discarded plaything—or is it flying, like an errant sea gull? It seems both friendly and ominous, implying that I am close to land. It wants to conquer me brutally, or to bring me gently into a larger world, I am not sure which. Then I awaken, shaking, and check the sheets again to see if they are damp.

I used to think that identity was like immunity. In some ways I still do. If only I could define myself, I think, I would be safe. I would have a secure perimeter I could defend. A territory, a turf, impenetrable even to a virus that pretended to belong to me, even a virus that does belong to me. I would be like Cuba, a homeland impossible to visit, proclaiming myself AIDS free, an island, my own world, with set boundaries and as yet unexplored interior mountains and jungles. A whole geography of its own to learn. I would be protected from outside influence, from the wars, diseases, and societal upheaval of other peoples. My revolution completed, the color of blood on my flag would have new, unexpected meanings.

No matter how much I fortify, however, AIDS seems to demand that I suffer too. It claims me. It is insistently part of my identity. At the very least, the pointed finger of epidemiology has singled me out. For once, I fit into too many categories. If money does talk, then its conversations about

AIDS have been busy awkwardly naming those of us who are most likely to get the disease. The powerful have been practicing saying out loud, if only briefly, those unmentionable people who are then otherwise ignored and remain oppressed, people who live what seem unimaginable lives: the drug addict we look away from as we pass her in the street, the son who has been disowned and kicked out of his home by his parents, the crack baby abandoned quivering in the incubator. We have said, with our newfangled antiretroviral vocabulary, that AIDS belongs to another people. Medicine for years said AIDS was a gay disease. Government waited several more years before a president said the word "AIDS" in public. Fundamentalist religion still implies AIDS is a punishment, meted out by an unloving, unforgiving, and unimaginable God, filled with wrath.

So I am grateful for the poetry that is written about AIDS, in that it has helped me so generously to locate myself in a world irrevocably altered by the presence of the virus. In contrast, the place where I went first for guidance—my medical education—at times steered me away from dealing with AIDS, even from working with AIDS patients. Harvard Medical School sometimes seemed better designed for attracting money for AIDS research than for preparing its students for the care of people with AIDS. Most of the time, it seemed a process invested in reassuring itself and its students that nothing had changed for the greater part of the world. I was taught early on how to be suspicious and how to inflict pain. I was shown slide after slide of schematic representations of the virus infecting nameless, faceless, unidentifiable cells. I was taught universal precautions, by the practice of which, I was led to imagine, the universe could be saved from what could only be understood as a grave threat to its, and my profession's, safety. I was armed with toxic drugs, because there had not been enough research yet to equip me with safer, more effective alternatives. I was even given an alter ego—as a future physician, I could not, by definition, be gay and only marginally and hardly noticeably Latino—and therefore I was protected. I was supplied with excuses for my inability to act—I was no longer personally involved. In fact, it was imperative that I keep a professional distance from my patients, so I could best serve them.

My own biases certainly colored my experience of medical school. I remained deeply conflicted about my choice of career and longed to have more time to write poetry. It was easy to blame medical school itself for my unhappiness. In fact, I used the inflexibility and rigor of medical school to contain what I thought of as my wild, unacceptable impulses. Perhaps, I imagined, Harvard could make me straight, an upstanding citizen, more American, less likely to have AIDS. Perhaps, by allowing myself to be distanced from people with AIDS, by doing research fifteen stories up in a monolithic concrete building dissecting rats' eyes under a microscope, I could improve my immunity, I could make myself blind to my connections to those dying people. If only I could take out my own eyes. If only I could trade in my poet's voice box for that newfangled, antiretroviral vocabulary, for a clean-cut physician's anatomically perfect larynx.

Moving to San Francisco from Boston, and from impressionable/repressed medical student to self-styled new resident, had a great impact on my perceptions of my training. Ward 5A (referred to knowingly as "5-AIDS" by the house staff in one of the hospitals where I worked) is the place where people with AIDS are cared for by a dedicated group of nurses, doctors, social workers, and volunteers. It was for me the most oddly familiar place of all the oddly familiar places in the hospital. Late at night, after restarting an IV or evaluating a new fever, I lingered in a patient's room to talk. Or, in one particular case, to read Thom Gunn's poetry aloud—when we heard the respirator functioning in the plunging up-and-down iambics of "Lament," we nearly cried together. I have mixed my voice with theirs. I have been fortunate to breathe in their sweet exhalations. I have, in fact, exchanged the same bodily secretions, albeit with others, but knowing somehow that all desire is the same. I may even have received the same person's blood by transfusion; ultimately, it is as though we were all from the same country.

In this spirit of connectedness, I thought once very briefly about teaching a poetry-writing workshop on the ward, during months when I would not be on call—before I realized that these people, my patients, have been teaching *me* to write all along. Speaking all the more clearly and rarely through their oxygen masks, they demonstrate to me the parallel yet opposing processes of victimization and creativity: to tell me the story of their lives, it strikes me painfully as I jot down my medical histories, is for them to become authors of their very destinies. The circumstances under which they live, threatened by declining health caused by a virus for which we are always reminded there is no cure, challenge them to remake their lives. Recounting the experience of sharing a needle, they have their hands on that needle again; they are existing before the virus entered their lives. They invent the cure with each narrative.

Indeed, they have taught me that when I write about AIDS, or about myself in relation to the virus, or about any patients' experiences, I am reinventing the medical history I am obliged to take. Facts become mere possibilities; in another version, the patient lives to see her grandchildren, and the painful memory of her dead husband who contracted AIDS from a prostitute is retold, so that the unfaithful one is reconstituted, somehow, as human and forgivable. Possibilities, in turn, are transformed into facts; all along, right under our noses, AZT, or colostrum, or six hours of hopeful meditation a day has been the miracle cure just waiting to be discovered. AIDS, in the process of rendering people almost unable to talk, filling lungs with secretions and opportunistic infections, has at the same time brought the same people to an opportunity for unmatchable eloquence, to retell their lives, to write the poems that will last forever in the troubled minds of future generations looking back on the epidemic.

I have thought that, perhaps, by knowing and caring for these men and women I might assume just a bit of the greatness embodied by them, brought to the brink of death in their presence by the disease. At my most honest and terrified moments, what I really hope to gain is some control over the wildly destructive force the virus has become. The kind of control that comes with being at peace with the prospect of one's death. I wrote a sonnet not long ago that I devised to be a sort of contraption, a spring-locked box—a tiny coffin for the AIDS virus— which I still reread, even now, whenever I am over- whelmed by seeing the faces of my patients, and by the unmistakable resemblance to my own face, over and over again, among those of people dying of AIDS. It is an unre- lenting, unforgiving love poem for a virus spread relent- lessly by acts of desire for love. A condom made of words that can be used in retrospect; or better yet, an entirely new world wherein sex is gloriously only sex—condoms, viruses, and coffins unheard of—a world without the care- ful calculations of one's risk and the imagined, deadly repercussions.

So-called formal poetry holds the most appeal for me because in it are present the fundamental beating contents of the body at peace: the regularity of resting brain wave activity in contrast to the disorganized spiking of a seizure, the gentle ebb and flow of breathing, or sobbing, in con- trast to the harsh spasmodic cough, the single-voiced, ringing chant of a slogan at an ACT UP rally in contrast to the indecipherable rumblings of AIDS-funding debate on the Senate floor. The poem is a physical process, is bodily exercise: rhymes become the mental resting places in the ascending rhythmic stairway of memory. The poem perhaps is an idealization, or a dream of the physical—the imagined healthy form. Yet it does not renounce illness; rather, it reinterprets it as the beginning point for healing.

I wonder, then, whether poetry might also be therapeutic. Many of my friends, especially my colleagues in medicine, have teased me for believing in the curative power of words, joking that I should write some doggerel on my prescriptions instead of the names of medications and directions for their use. If poetry is made of breath, or the beating heart, then surely it is not unreasonable to think it might reach those places in the bodies of its audience, however rarefied. Moreover, I joke back, I have never seen a poem cause fulminant liver failure or bone marrow toxicity, even a really bad one. Putting the mouth to words, and by incantation returning regular rhythms to the working lungs, these were the principles by which ancient healers in Native American cultures practiced their art. The Egyptians gave their dead a book full of charms and spells to be used in the afterlife—might not poetry, then, facilitate the passing to another realm? Poetry is a pulsing, organized imagining of what once was, or is to be. What life once was, what life is to be. It is ampules of the purest, clearest drug of all, the essence and distillation of the process of living itself.

I do not deny that most of the interventions Western medicine makes available to AIDS patients have their basis in scientific principles and truths, to the best that we can determine what those truths might be. I have delivered aggressive care to people with AIDS. I can compare the feeling of placing an endotracheal tube in a patient in respiratory distress only to the feeling of writing about the experience afterward. A twenty-eight-year-old man most likely would have died before our eyes had it not been for that tube. It was our explicit objective, after conferring as much as possible with him given the acuity of the situation, to save his life; he indicated that he wished to be intubated. As we sedated him (because he still contained so much life at that critical moment that he was able to fight the respirator), I watched his face change. He had lost his language: the endotracheal tube by anatomical necessity passes through the vocal cords in connecting the respirator to the airspaces of the lungs, thereby taking away one's ability to speak.

I am still not sure whether what he needed more during those last few days of his life was to speak or to breathe. The pneumonia that had made it so difficult for him to breathe on his own progressed rapidly, despite the various "big gun" antibiotics we infused into his veins. His fever climbed. We had given him a chance to live longer, reinstituting, if clumsily, the natural rhythm of breathing—had he survived the massive infection, the tube might have eventually come out—but it was at the cost of his last words. He died without last words. His parents flew in from New Jersey the night before he died, called in by his lover. They had not spoken in ten years, since the day he had told them he was gay and they threw him out in a rage. His mother stayed up all night, singing lullabies to him, comforting him, and perhaps herself, with small verses so familiarly rhymed. Hearing them comforted me too. When his blood pressure began to fall, quite suddenly, I imagined that his soul had already begun its departure, leaving his body only partly filled with the physical ingredients of life left behind, like powder in a loose sack. I imagined his soul, dancing away upon the rise and fall of his mother's quiet voice, each syllable a timid, graceful footfall.

Sometime later, perhaps weeks after he died, I heard his voice speak to me. It was in the form of a poem. The respirator and the lullaby were keeping time in the background, but what I heard most distinctly was his voice. He was breathing on his own again, and his breathing had taken on the quality of flight. Lying in my own bed, dreaming my dream of infinite blood, I imagined opening my eyes and seeing him standing naked before me. His entire body seemed to pulse with the poem he was creating. He was naming his body; his body was extremely beautiful, and I noticed every tiny imperfection, and cared deeply and attentively about it, as he spoke about the afterlife. It was as though he had left these words unspoken, and now they flowed over me so effortlessly that I could almost understand them. I could almost understand a death caused by AIDS.

When I began writing about AIDS myself, I felt I was returning some of those words to the world. So much is unspoken—AIDS is not just a forbidden subject in most circles, it is absolutely unthinkable. Now when I see SILENCE = DEATH painted on the sidewalk, or pinned to the lapel of my white coat, immediately I know what that means. It means our words *are* keeping us alive. Our words are the currency of our existence, the funds we spend to fight the disease, the blood spilled in the demonstrations, the tears shed and the semen ejaculated by and for our lovers. When I read Thom Gunn, or Marilyn Hacker, or Paul Monette, or Assoto Saint, I am hearing this unthinkable but fiercely inhabited voice. A voice that wishes not simply to reclaim the body but to celebrate it. A voice that desires fearlessly, without risks. A voice that heals. A voice from behind the respirator, from behind a mother's lips.

In ravaging our collective immunity, in literally wearing its victims down to the bone, AIDS by its very existence makes the naked body that much more clearly delineated; it is almost like beholding a person in the last stages of the disease. The spoken word becomes that much more urgent and honest, the poem that much more purely language. When addressing AIDS, the poet him/herself is no longer immune to the outer world, to its biases and hate. Before the blank page, I have felt myself to be utterly available, and this form of freedom is the hardest part, because it is the most terrifying freedom there is. The poetry of AIDS, then, is not simply and always about assuming control. Rewritten: it is about losing all control, about dying and fucking. Souls dissolving into songs, memories of a lost lover last seen in New Orleans, laments.

Sometimes I look to their bodies for a definitive answer to my ongoing prayer for understanding. I remember how I felt when I touched my grandfather's scars, those deep imprints left by Cuba: I was a blind child reading the past in Braille, understanding for the first time the vast planta-

tion, the raging river, the cattle, the dark jail, and the soldiers' clubs. When I ask my patients to undress, I think of
him. I touch the skin, feel the texture, the warmth of a new
purple spot. I examine the breast, collect a bit of the dis-
charge. The heart sounds always seem louder, more
urgent, but I wonder whether that is because so many have
already lost so much weight, their hearts only barely
beneath the surface. I listen to the abdomen, digesting
everything, the internal, constant interface with the outside world. I try desperately not to desire them, because it
is unprofessional, and because it is too human and scary
and powerful. I imagine having their bodies, though, pos-
sessing them as I do my own, occupying that same space.
It feels exactly the same, except perhaps it is more wonderful to be naked (even in the air-conditioned, too metal-
lic office the hospital provides me). Maybe I am only
feeling free of my usual armor, my needle hands and ophthalmoscope eyes transformed into soft fingers and gentle,
green irises. Funny how I never feel the pain, though I can
often reproduce it in them as I press and poke the indicated region. Pain must be too personal, held too deeply with
the body, to be known without actually experiencing it.
Though my grandfather's smile emphasized a certain scar
on his forehead, and therefore could feel like a blow to the
head, so bitter and full of loss, I never felt the pain he must
have known. I can only imagine it.

Seeing their bodies makes me remember a priest's ser-
mon I heard when I was a small child in Venezuela. A
blinding white church, all right angles, dusty, vibrant heat,

red-tiled floor, roughly hewn wooden pews that might give you a splinter. It was a eulogy of sorts. He was asking us to imagine Christ's suffering on the cross. How willing we all were, closing our eyes tightly, driving the nails through our hands and feet, allowing the spear into our livers, the air conditioner humming as we sat enraptured, silent. Was I willing to die for my sins? For the sins of others? I wondered at the common experience of imagining such pain and suffering. I wondered whether people were really feeling Christ's wounds, or whether like me they were recalling to their minds the times when they had cut themselves with a sharp knife they should not have been using in the first place, or fell off a bicycle—or, since they were mostly women, whether they were remembering their breast cancer surgery or their husbands' beating them. Some *viejitas* up in front began moaning gently, then sobbing. The spell was broken suddenly when the priest loudly scolded us: *No!* he shouted, Christ's suffering was a mystery and utterly unknowable. Only through faith could we achieve redemption, and it was the relief of pain through God's forgiveness that was to be our eternal reward in heaven. As he became more and more animated, his voice rising toward indignation and anger and salvation, I lost myself staring at the emaciated peeling figure above the altar, crucified for the benefit of our eyes and souls. I have lost myself the same way in the faces, the bodies, and the poems of people with AIDS. I see them teaching us, each one of us, the meaning of our own losses. Teaching us that every word is true.

Nor Are We Immune:
A Poet's Manifesto ⌒

After these sixty-five died, the Indians of that country came down with a
stomach ailment that killed half their people. They thought that we were
the cause of their deaths. . . .
       —*Cabeza de Vaca, from "The Account"*

Is it fear of death with which I'm so eager
to live my life out

now and in its possible permutations
with the one I love?
       —*Marilyn Hacker, from "Late November"*

He was dying even then, as I hurried away from the ICU on my way to the noontime conference. It was the end of the academic year, that time when all the senior residents were giving their formal talks. These swan songs were each usually preceded by an awkward introduction by our white-haired program director, often over the clamor of an overworked and unruly audience of house staff helping itself to the complimentary lunch provided by some smiling, sparklingly polished drug company rep. Invariably, these introductions would demonstrate how little the administration cared to know about the nervous speaker, as names were mispronounced, alma maters misidentified, and flattering adjectives fumbled. I squeezed through the crowded maze of chairs to a seat off to the side of the narrow room, almost against the back wall.

Sitting down with my plate heaped full of mushy tortellini, I paused to admire the shiny new pen to which I had also been treated, which advertised the name of a newly patented (and therefore extremely expensive) antibiotic for the therapy of community-acquired pneumonia and other common infections. Another cheap pen: I never dared to presume I might someday use it, like so many others distributed at such conferences, to write about AIDS, to record this small part of the unending story I am finally writing down now. At the time, maybe I was still waiting for the day when one of these drug reps would come with news of a great breakthrough in the treatment of AIDS, the disease that held my patient hostage in the ICU, whom I thought of once again, briefly and guiltily, as I stuffed the first forkful of pasta into my mouth in an effort to keep it occupied.

The lights dimmed then, and I was surprised to see displayed on the screen at the front of the conference room the first slide: a sixteenth-century rendering of Taino indians in various stages of a disease that was killing them. The depiction of the savages was grotesque. Their skin was pock-marked with blistering lesions. Their backs were covered with hair and their heads shaved, and their bodies were contorted and bowed in the presence of not only the visible Europeans but also their more formidable invisible microbes. For the next hour, instead of something like the more typical clinically oriented topics of past weeks—"Update on Colon Cancer" or "Strategies for the Management of Peptic Ulcer Disease"—we learned about the effect of diseases brought by these European explorers upon indigenous New World populations, and the dramatic impact these diseases had on history by effectively facilitating the brutal conquest that ensued. I struggled to remain awake and even alert for the entire talk, which was remarkable given that I was post-call and would normally have nodded off right after gobbling up my free lunch, having slept only two or three fitful hours during the previous night.

The speaker's relatively few comments with regards to AIDS, however, were far less enlightening than the greater portion of his talk. Though he spoke with pained eloquence about the tragedy of the wholesale destruction of Native Americans at the hands of his own ancestors, he seemed unable to draw any parallels between what had happened in the past and what was going on all around us. He essentially dismissed the AIDS epidemic as a relatively trivial phenomenon as compared with smallpox or dysentery. Smallpox had been in some instances deliberately transmitted to Native Americans, he explained, and certainly was in no way behaviorally transmitted among these innocent, simple people; furthermore, smallpox had wiped out innumerable specific cultures in the period of a single century. AIDS, on the other hand, was affecting only relatively small and marginalized groups of people in present-day America, whose behaviors were largely responsible for transmitting the disease that afflicted them.

The more he said, the more profoundly mute I seemed to become. My mind flashed once again to my patient in the ICU, dying by degrees so inexorably, silenced so violently by the rigid plastic tube roughly inserted through his vocal cords and into his trachea, one of the 50 percent of gay men in San Francisco who are HIV positive or living with AIDS. I knew he would never speak again. Surely, the telling of stories and the bellowing of poetry are requisite for the maintenance and evolution of a culture, I thought; when the languages of Native Americans have vanished, almost without exception so have their own, perhaps more accurate versions of their histories. All that remains of them is the distorted images and tall tales left behind by the victors.

Internally, I tried to make some sense of this earnest white man's account of a set of events neither of us had witnessed, but which he recounted with such calm assurance. Having stood blinking in the quiet surrounding so many failed resuscitations, I knew that to lose one's own voice was indeed tantamount to death. Inevitably, I began to reflect upon what I had long ago come to view as the problem of my own writing. My poetry, the two slim volumes that exist and that seem so puny an effort in the face of the richness of intersecting queer and Latino cultures, long suffered under my own efforts to repress it, for fear. Fear that it was too small, fear that it was not manly enough, fear that it might somehow betray my secrets or

the location of my hideout to my potential enemies, fear
that my linguistic mannerisms or my invisible accent or my
misuse of grammar might embarrass me, fear that I might
become the property or the exotic pet of the rich white
people who want to help, fear of any such help itself.
Reenacting the countless stifled poems I never wrote, and
still may never write, I have stopped myself from crying at
the bedside of a dying patient, squelched my retort on
rounds when a homophobic comment is thoughtlessly
dropped. I admit that I once aspired to insiderliness, entering through the back doors and taking the service eleva-
tors of grand institutions like Amherst and Harvard; I also
confess that I have censored myself willingly, like so many
writers who are finally (no matter where they shop or
whom they sleep with) outside of the mainstream—but
never without recognizing, however distantly, a great cost
to my sense of merit, of usefulness, of equality, of pride.

Understanding this process may be the only way to
obviate it, but understanding required at that moment a
sustained level of energy and concentration that was beginning to elude me. I began to daydream more deeply,
instead, about the possibility of a kind of homosexual country of origin, a different and fabulously free New World, a
place whose existence seemed plausible to me after so
many long and tortured journeys I had made across oceans
of disavowal to the deepest reaches of my heart. On each
of these journeys, a vast and unexplored continent
stretched before me there, in the shape of a man's body. I
had the feeling that I was searching for something of

tremendous value. A people inhabited the land, a people not unlike the Tainos, the Choctaws, or the Mayans in that they were peaceful, highly intelligent, and tolerant of relationships between members of the same sex. These people, though possessed of a clear sense of identity, were faceless to me, and their immune systems apparently functioned differently. They were as naked to the microbes of hate and inhumanity as their bodies were to me. They had incredibly long eyelashes, and their eyes were sea green. They disregarded the ample evidence that significant quantities of gold, silver, and gemstones lay beneath the surface of their land, which itself, I hated to admit, was beautiful.

Though I too wished to strip off my clothes, shed my immunity, and make love to one of their men beneath the warm sun as I noticed my skin becoming more brown, something kept preventing me. What was it? I spoke a different language, I wanted to convert them to Catholicism, I wanted to translate their poetry to fit my own interpretations, and I wanted their gold. Before long, I developed the overpowering urge to obliterate them. So it always is upon the first contact with the unknown. My mind was flooded with so many unbelievable stories I wanted to invent about them, stories that in their telling would make them belong to me. At the same time, I wanted to re-create them in my own image, the image of what existed in the culture of violence and hatred I knew I could never leave behind.

So I devised a plan, involving a new disease that affected only African slaves and thus was little understood. I knew they would not be naturally protected against it; during my brief time among them, I had observed that they became ill and died with exposure to the most trivial and common of diseases. Since my background was in medicine, it would furthermore be an interesting experiment in the pathogenesis of a terminal illness, and would provide at the same time the opportunity to discredit their own approaches to healing. Perhaps I would become famous and have the most renowned laboratory in the world. Best of all, it was a disease transmitted by sexual contact, and so my preaching to them about the ungodliness of fornication and the possibility of redemption in the Savior would be reinforced with a most deadly vehemence.

One of them, a young chieftain, tried to speak with me, not knowing what I had planned. His language seemed to emanate from his heart and was therefore hypnotic. I stared into his green eyes, admiring his long, girlish eyelashes. The sun pressed down upon us, with a weight I could liken only to a great grief. I realized that inexplicably I was falling in love with him, which made it all the more difficult to infect him. Just as our lips were about to touch, just when I thought for the thousandth time that I would finally be able to pinpoint exactly where I was, a dim alarm sounded from far away. The high, piercing tone sounded terribly familiar, but I was too deeply lost somewhere in my heart to orient myself correctly, lost irretrievably as I was in the densest of jungles. . . .

When the annoyed resident sitting next to me shook my arm, I realized the noise in my dream was my beeper going off, and we were already in the question-and-answer period of the talk. I was not sure how long I had been asleep, but my confusion promptly evaporated when I saw the telephone number to which I had been summoned: it was the ICU! I bolted out of my chair and raced down the infinitely long hallway to the familiar set of mechanized doors, which made their insatiably hungry sucking noise as they opened before me, admitting me once again to what each day seemed more and more like a spaceship of modern medicine. Finally at his bedside, I saw in the pulsing monitors and readouts that he was hypotensive and tachycardic, very near the brink of death.

We had been having trouble ventilating him since his first day in the unit; it was his fourth bout of pneumocystis pneumonia, which this time had caused complete whiteout of both lungs, and he remained hypoxemic despite the administration of 100 percent oxygen. His partner huddled with his parents, and they all stood by the bedside crying softly, courageously defying to be drawn into the vortex of his downward spiral. I barked out a few orders; miraculously, after some fluids and the initiation of low-dose dopamine, his blood pressure drifted upward and his heart rate came down, so that both were hovering within the near-normal range. I had the distinct sense that he had weathered a force as powerful as any hurricane, and that he had been saved without too much undue suffering, only to lie wrecked upon the shoreline of that same distant and deserted land in my heart. As I looked upon his fiercely handsome face, still handsome despite its gradual and relentless effacement by AIDS, despite the plastic tube taped at an angle securely to his delicate cheekbone, I noticed as though for the first time his long eyelashes, fluttering over his sea green eyes.

I came home that night, exhausted, and intensively began to write again for the first time in many months. I felt compelled to respond to the opposing themes at play in this sequence of interactions, motifs omnipresent in my life since I committed myself to a career in the healing arts: greed and generosity, imperialism and non-nationness, silence and voice, medicine and poetry, reality and fantasy, disease and immunity, genocide and identity. As I put pen to paper, I felt again boiling in my own blood the conflicts between the heavily armored Spaniards and Englishmen whose tongues still have expression in my own brain, and the debilitated and diseased Indians whose darker coloration has barely survived in my own skin. Enslaved by my own ancestors, and alienated from my own profession, I wondered again whether my words would in fact be of use to anyone. Made ostensibly powerless by an incomprehensible disease—and with the horizons of my impotence extending in all directions, from inescapable guilt for having escaped (so far) HIV infection myself, to nagging ambivalence regarding the falsely reassuring exhortations about safe sex coming from the medical profession, to an enforced speechlessness as a queer culture as multifaceted and invaluable as any of those of the Native Americans that were destroyed during the conquest of the New World disintegrates before my very eyes—how could I continue to respond merely with morphine and pressors, but not their attendant poetry, to another person dying of AIDS?

To help answer this question, I must continue to excavate my experiences of medical school, a place that I inhabited fearfully, at a time of many transitions for me and the profession. I recall vividly my sense early in my training that identity was somehow intertwined with immunity; that the two words rhyme has always suggested to me a secret but certain relationship. The early empirical data I gathered made me think that those people who knew what or who they were manifested a magical protection against disease. On the other hand, it was those who were marginalized and splintered who seemed especially susceptible to illness. What I observed led me to postulate for myself a Theorem of Health: The fellowship of man conferred resistance to disease, while selfishness and alienation induced it. Now I understand that this distinction I perceived—the class and race distinctions between the people who more commonly die of their diseases and those who do not—is grounded upon the fragmentation of the communities of those who are outnumbered, the differentially more limited access they have to health care, the bias they suffer in the delivery of care, the differences in levels of education they can attain, and other confounding parameters that reflect economic and political disenfranchisement. But back then, all I knew was that the poor patients said very little and almost never asked questions.

At that formative moment, I also tried to decipher the riddle of my own body's insistence on living. My own state of relatively good health seemed at odds with my feelings of isolation. I began to contemplate myself as a potential locus for the diseases I was learning about, imagining a strange and particular pathophysiology at work among my genetically discordant cells. I needed to belong to some single category, some easily defined group, yet two sexes seemed to dwell inside me, providing twice as many opportunities for diseases to take root; I wondered whether internally I might have twice as many organs, whether I contained a rudimentary uterus and pair of ovaries lying dormant in the depths of my body and giving rise to my "unnatural" desires. My immune system, I worried as my eczema worsened, in attempting to distinguish self from nonself as it combed over the most intimate crevices of my every cell, might be finding some exotic protein marker in the skin I inherited from my Cuban grandparents unacceptable, and was initiating a process of rejection that would lead to the autoimmune destruction of my lungs, my larynx, my entire being. Every surface, every orifice, every dark place where organs functioned, all were the potential points of entry for my eventual unmaking, a process in which I was complicit because of who I was—or was not. It was in this way that medicine provided for me a method for pathologizing myself, a way to confirm what it had been telling me in other ways since I had first considered a career in medicine: that I did not belong, and that I was not welcome. That I was *unhealthy*. I heard my profession's message of reproach in the same language that we both spoke, using the same exclusionary terms, to the very people we were supposed to be helping.

Despite these impending sicknesses of mine, I could consider myself fortunate at least in one respect: I was amazed each time I realized how one of my patients was caring for me, providing me the comfort and reassurance that my own profession often denied me as I attempted to battle disease, especially AIDS. They, the infirm and dying, were my unlikely support group. Even as my patients grew more and more ill, even as their bodies grew more and more crowded with opportunistic pathogens, they still found room in their hearts to keep me safe. Their goodwill sometimes seemed inexhaustible, even when they were faced with the ongoing belligerence so many of them encountered as they negotiated their way through the labyrinthine X ray suites, laboratories, hospitals, and pharmacies of the medical otherworld. They shared their narratives with me guardedly at first, unsure whether they would have the time to finish telling them; they seemed so painfully baffled that they should go on living for years with a disease that everyone, especially so many physicians, insisted was fatal.

Such generosity made no sense to me even until recently. I had self-importantly taught myself to conceive of caring for people with AIDS in almost punitive terms, akin to giving a kicking, screaming child a shot: I hated to do it, but I had to. I remember reacting with this exact combination of distaste and resignation when a young Latino man named Manuel first came to my office, after I had weathered medical school and become a lowly intern. He had the dark mestizo features shared by many of my Mexican American patients, but sported a black leather motorcycle jacket and a pink-triangle earring, and at first his self-assured manner made me hope privately that he might be just a healthy gay man coming in for a routine physical, and I was eager to create the comfortable and accepting environment I had never felt when visiting physicians myself. I quickly learned that Manuel was not interested in his own comfort, however. After a few polite introductory questions and answers, he proceeded to tell me bluntly of the fifty to possibly one hundred anonymous sexual encounters with other men he had engaged in over the past few months, all in a concerted effort to become infected with HIV. He wanted to contract AIDS.

He seemed so sure of who he was, he seemed so proud a member of his communities, and yet this confident self was what he wanted to destroy. I could barely hide my fast-rising disgust and rage, while a less emotional part of me bristled with disbelief. He kept talking anyway, perhaps sensing some remnant in me that was still capable of listening. He wanted to die, he said, because he could not stand to wipe up another lover's diarrhea from the floor in a dining room where they had once shared meals with other friends long since dead of AIDS; he could not bear another message from his mother on his answering machine wondering whether he was still alive, imploring him to leave San Francisco and return to their church in the Central Valley. He had come to believe that HIV infection was as inevitable as seeing his own face in the mirror when he shaved in the morning, as much a part of his life as attending memorial services and reading the obituaries. He would not let himself become another victim, he said, but rather would face his destiny with courage. He paused and looked me dead in the eye.

I felt a weight beginning to shift in my chest, as though a new passageway were being pried open. Here was a man my age who seemed to embody fully his various identities better than I knew the uncannily similar ones that were my own, and yet he was actually courting the disease I had been drafted into fighting. My pat theories about health and disease ran away from me as I stared back into his unclouded face. When I checked off the box on the appropriate blue lab form, for a moment I too hoped his blood test would come back positive, that the antibodies would be found in his bloodstream, to show that at least his body was fighting the infection, even if psychologically he had accepted it, and had already succumbed. In that moment of wordless connection, I realized as if for the first time that I too had wanted to die for so long and for so many reasons myself, out of guilt for being HIV negative, out of my old self-loathing for being gay in the first place, out of the strange wish for the washed-out whiteness the anemia caused by antiretrovirals might create in my own olive complexion. I shut off my thinking by blankly repeating for the thousandth time the meaning of a positive test (HIV only present in the blood, but not equivalent to the diagnosis of AIDS), and what negative meant (does not rule out exposure to HIV). Manuel laughed when I insisted he sign on the dotted line indicating his understanding and his consent to undergo the test, and joked that he could have done a better job counseling himself.

To my astonishment, despite my antipathy and ineptitude, Manuel returned dutifully two weeks later, so eager was he to learn the results of his test. I suspected he had been through this sequence of events so many times before that it had become second nature. When, trembling, I read out the positive results, his unexpected smile of relief collided with my reflexive hopelessness. I could bear his smugness and determination no longer; I demanded to know why he seemed so happy. His gentle shrug of acceptance only heightened my distress. Before I could come to my senses, he left abruptly, thanking me for my help but without telling me how I could possibly go on. He never returned.

For a time, I wondered what happened to Manuel, whether he sought out the help of a more expert physician, or whether he simply returned to Fresno after all, where perhaps he would help educate young people about AIDS before dying surrounded by his family. I wondered whether he went back to the dark sex clubs to infect others as desperately fed up as he was, or whether he became an activist who distributed pamphlets and condoms outside their doors. I wondered whether he would ever speak out publicly about his experiences, about the kind of remorse and desolation of the spirit that could lead to the form of suicide he chose; I wondered whether he went home to an apartment in the Castro full of books and ghosts, a room full of haunting yet comforting poetry that might sing him to sleep. Ultimately, I resented him for what I judged he had done to himself. Curing for me had for so long taken precedence over caring: assigning individual people to neat categories in order to risk-stratify them, over getting to know my patients. Dr. Anthony Fauci's clinical pronouncements in *Science* took precedence over the complex wisdom in the poetry of June Jordan or Thom Gunn. I had yet to understand why anyone might decline to be immune, or how poetry might embody the *refusal* to be saved.

I continue to hear from my colleagues, and oftentimes from my own mouth, the automatic refrain that has been our primary response to the epidemic thus far: safe sex, safe sex, safe sex, two seductively alliterative words that would drown out all the true poetry. Yet I am beginning to believe that this approach, besides doing little to prevent transmission of the AIDS virus, because mottos are far less effective barriers than actual latex, may in fact be counterproductive. These days, it seems I daily encounter patients much like Manuel in my clinical practice—and many others like my patient in the ICU, who could never express it to me as directly—whose response to the safe-sex, "Be Here for the Cure" message has been essentially one of hopelessness and, paradoxical as it might seem, *lack* of control. Many still see such catchphrases, and the numerous other related ill-conceived (however well-intentioned) campaigns they have spawned, as simply an echo from a black and possibly bottomless chasm. The diversity of expression, the richness of response possible only through the discourse of poetry and human connection, is flattened by each new bumper sticker. The ailing body politic no longer feverishly throbs and swells, but instead is cut off, sterilized, devitalized, and chastened. Almost as nullifying as silence itself, the sanitary images and nice bland words we can say in public that seem to be the engines of the public health establishment's representation of AIDS seem to have backfired on all of us. In their place, I have found myself wishing that more poems would be written, in red graffiti spray-painted across vacant billboards—that more rules be broken, that the truth be told.

A growing number of people in the communities most devastated by AIDS want to surrender. Cerebrally, we all know that AIDS can kill us, and yet willfully some are choosing not to be immune and not to speak out. Particularly among young gay men, who are coming out and establishing their identities in the context of such overwhelming numbers of casualties in a war that must appear to them impossible to win—over ten thousand AIDS deaths by January 1994 in San Francisco alone, the vast majority of them gay men, and disproportionately people of color—I have continued to hear expressed the desire to become infected with HIV, to "get it over with." Instead of the gorgeous elegy, in place of the defiant war cry, I hear in them the grim parody of safe-sex slogans, just as curt, just as unfeeling. Oftentimes these startling death wishes come in the wake of a particular friend's, or ex-part-ner's, or role model's recent death from AIDS. Safe-sex messages directed *exclusively* at young gay men not only single them out and isolate them further but also suggest a terrible conflation of falling in love, or even of simply being gay, with disease, death, and loss. Their desire, then, for death underscores how little I and my medical profession have had to offer these understandably frightened, grief-stricken, and confused young people.

So when critics of AIDS education point to the alarming rise in new cases of HIV infection among young gay men as proof of the failure of these efforts, demanding funding cuts and censoring already too insipid public health campaigns, the irony becomes so painfully clear that it is difficult not to imagine that a conscious strategy is being quite successfully employed. The efforts of such hate mongers to define AIDS as an exclusively homosexual disease, and therefore to limit government expenditures to combat its spread, have dovetailed nicely with the efforts of AIDS activists to utilize most effectively their paucity of funds to hammer upon those perceived to be at highest risk of HIV infection; by so narrowly defining their target group, educators end up fulfilling the most delirious prophecies of their enemies. The unidimensional doomsaying only serves to heighten the guilt, hopelessness, fear of (and loss of pleasure in) sex, powerlessness, judgment-impairing substance abuse, and denial—all expected responses of any group of people witnessing its own ongoing annihilation.

The four newest seroconversions in the past several months of three young gay men and an African American

woman in my practice, to whom all I had to say as recorded in my clinic progress notes was "safe-sex practices discussed and reinforced," could sadly testify to this fact.
Efforts to interrupt the cycle that leads to the ongoing
transmission of AIDS might focus instead on the psychological sequelae of surviving in the wide-open jaws of
death, and not just upon attacking in a generalized manner
the supposedly risky behaviors that many consider integral
to sexual identity. Helping individuals to understand such
self-destructive impulses as might exist in them, in the
context of complete and more accurate information about
behaviors that transmit the AIDS virus, would likely save
more lives than millions of glossy brochures mindlessly
espousing "safe sex."

I have in the past resisted the simplistic notion that what
I do in bed primarily defines my overall identity as a person. I resented the assumptions that because I was gay, I
was not man enough to become a physician, that I was
doomed never to enjoy the romance of falling in love and
forming a stable long-term committed relationship, that I
rejected all the teachings of my religion, that I would be so
unfulfilled that I might someday be driven to commit suicide, that I could write only sissified and thus worthless
poetry, that I would someday die of AIDS. So I went off to
medical school and became a physician, I met a man who
will always be the love of my life, I have maintained an
interrogatory faith in God, and I have neither killed myself
nor died of AIDS—and none of these seem, despite the
upheavals along the way, surprising in the least. I have

even kept writing, a thin book of poems hidden in my back pocket, in spite of myself. So the specific experience of having another man's cock inside my mouth, or having mine inside another man's rectum, had to be trivial, totally irrelevant.

In the face of the AIDS crisis, however, such physical expressions of love have become revolutionary indeed, as revolutionary and as physical for me as the act of writing poetry. Some might call them unpatriotic, even traitorous and punishable by death. Like the "illegal aliens" who penetrate the forbidden border of this country desperate for the chance at a better life, and who remain the objects (in California especially) of one of the most venomous campaigns ever conceived to protect American national integrity—and, incidentally, to prevent their access to public education, heath care, and other costly services—I can see that I too have been transformed into an otherworldly being. Ironically, the Native Americans welcomed their strange visitors from Europe, providing them with sustenance and shelter, often worshiping them as god-like figures; they were repaid with genocide, and the few survivors were dispossessed of their lands and the remnants of their cultures. Now some of the prosperous heirs of those who killed and enslaved have gone on to resurrect these practices in their responses not only to AIDS and undocumented immigration but also to health care reform and countless other issues. Whatever fortified and prohibited border it is that we violate, whether it is crossing the imaginary line that divides the United States from Mexico or

Haiti, or enjambing a line break too suggestively, or passing through the portal of the eroticized anus of a lesbian
or gay man, someone must necessarily stand accused.

That accusation is as audible in the safe-sex mantra as it
is heard on the floor of the U.S. Senate. It was present for
a long time in my own encounters with queer patients, and
certainly contributed to my own sense of despair in dealing with AIDS—until I realized that our sexual acts are
among the few scraps of identity that we do own, that we
must own. The kiss that locates us on a map of the known
world, the interlocking legs that are the sextant pointing
the way home, the renewing embrace that does not transmit HIV—even if they do not make up our identities
entirely, we must give them to ourselves freely and without remorse or encumbrances. If they are to continue the
struggle to stop AIDS, young gay people and people of
color must view themselves as pluripotent and vital, and
not simply as the next powerless victims, mopping up their
lovers' shit or intubated and voiceless in the ICU. They
need to know that they will write the poems that will survive, the breathtaking accounts that future generations will
look back on with astonishment and gratitude; they need
to enjoy sex, and not fear their erotic nature.

Happily, hope is beginning to be nurtured in a growing
number of writing workshops both for people living with
AIDS and for all of us who are the survivors of those who
have died, perhaps providing novel pathways away from
the possibility of new infection. I often wonder what
might have happened to Manuel if he had found his way

into one of them and had I met him sitting in a small circle in the basement of a community center, instead of across the desk in my institutionally drab medical office. I wonder whether he would have been moved by the story of my patient holding on in the ICU; I wonder whether he could have imagined a less perilous personal voyage, one that led not to a romance with death, which in the end could never replace those denied in life, but to a different, life-sustaining intimacy with another who shared his pain. I wonder if together we could have conjured up a cure for AIDS, blissfully unaware of the presumptuousness of such a notion, as we sipped bad coffee from Styrofoam cups. I wonder whether he might have fallen in love with someone who could have become his reason to live, to whom he would dedicate his poems.

Just as poetry might be of indispensable use to people living with AIDS and those who care for them, so might poetry find renewed purpose and vigor as it is reclaimed by those who are suffering and surviving. Too many poems in recent times have been written for the intimate, exclusive audience of other poets. In losing sight of the body from which they arise, this brand of poetry seems afraid to become sullied with the bodily secretions that carry the virus, afraid of the stubborn stain of blood, ashamed of the red letter of sex and passion. Poetry itself might learn a lesson from AIDS.

Even if it is not the miracle cure, the brave, heartfelt poem just might be the safest and most pleasurable sex of all, providing the kind of empowerment that comes from fully occupying one's body. It is the private space where the rhythms of ecstatic lovemaking can be felt without barriers. It is the place where anything can be said, where nothing like it has ever before been imagined; it is the bright laboratory where the virus is isolated, understood, and cured. It is what gets into your blood and makes you feel so robustly alive; it is the rhyme that returns you to childhood and makes you young again. It is the accumulated wisdom of the ancient healers who called upon Apollo and his lyre to restore his supplicants to health, and it recalls the percussive chants of the medicine men; it is all the rage and passion of Marilyn Hacker, the bitter tears of Mark Doty. It is felt in the heart, in the genitals, in the mouth and tongue. The poem just might contain the elusive secret formula to life itself.

At the same time we restore pleasurable sex to queer identity, and the pleasurable poem to the whole world's vocabulary, we must be cautious and more responsible in our efforts to educate our young people about AIDS, with particular attention to the psychological toll the disease continues to take on all members of the communities at risk. Besides advocating in a sex-positive light the use of condoms and oral-vaginal and oral-anal barriers *in settings where transmission is likeliest,* those at little risk of new exposure to HIV—that is, couples in monogamous relationships with both members of the same serostatus (positive or negative), couples engaging in mutual masturbation and insertive or receptive fellatio (the research on which indicates extremely low transmission rates), those who choose

to refrain from sexual activity, those who enjoy autoeroti-
cism—should be spared, as all of us should, the overt mor-
alizing that too often has characterized our approach thus
far and that only leads to the kind of hopelessness, substance abuse, and poor self-image that in turn results in the
type of deliberate (and almost deliberate) exposures I have
witnessed. The profound truth, so readily understood by
the rest of society at large, is simply this: not only is intimacy possible and pleasurable, but it is protective, renewing, even joyous, and ultimately liberating. Sex *is* safe, and
one of the most compelling reasons to avoid HIV is so one
can keep doing it.

We must also ceaselessly reeducate ourselves as to the
meaning of the presence of antibodies to HIV in the bloodstream. HIV-positive individuals should no longer be
viewed as living under a death sentence, nor have they
been punished for past behaviors or for not having practiced "safe sex." Instead, celebrating the lives of those who
are living proof that AIDS is not universally fatal is crucial,
and certainly not as "delusional" as some of the adversaries
of people with AIDS would like us to believe. Our approach
to maintaining the health of these people must be multidis-
ciplinary, with an effort to break down barriers among
providers in the same way we fight barriers to AIDS visi-
bility. Looking to other realms outside of traditional
Western medicine, with its sometimes toxic pharmacologic
agents and never-ending research protocols, to the other
complementary healing professions should not just be permissible but encouraged. The needs of all providers who

care for those living with AIDS—the psychologists, nurses, physicians, acupuncturists, pharmacists, chiropractors, spiritual healers, physician assistants, dentists, homeopaths, physical therapists, and, most important, families, friends, and lovers of people with AIDS—must also be addressed. The strengths of these potential alliances are too formidable for us to continue to squander them.

All those who see the terrible beauty in AIDS must dare to defy the odds. They must go on living, to be our wise and patient guides, to be our healers. As Manuel might have said, in a stunning poem that out-argued death—if only he had known that he needed to write it and we needed to hear it—we can still have the last word on AIDS. As my patient in the ICU might have said—removing the tube from his trachea and casting it aside, in the voice I never heard again miraculously restored—no AIDS death can be the burden any individual person must bear. This disease is our smallpox, our infected blanket that both kills us and keeps us warm; it is forever a chapter of our undying history. AIDS has taken far too many lives already, while we waited for that new antibiotic or antiretroviral. To know its power to change us, and to know what we must finally do to end its tyranny, we need only to look at one another, because the cure is etched indelibly in poetry upon our own enduring bodies.

Imagining
Unmanaging
Health Care ⁓

When I pretended during my early youth what it might be like to practice medicine, I did not dream of the satiny images and pearly white smiles from the Marcus Welby reruns I faithfully watched on television, nor did I fantasize about getting behind the wheel of the gleaming cherry red Mercedes convertible my uncle the psychiatrist drove to my family's frequent gatherings. Money and medicine, though somehow clearly linked, were to me incalculably unrelated. The power of doctors rested in their ability to heal the human beings in whom they recognized themselves wherever they touched them, not in making inanimate gold from their well-insured patients' flesh. The legendary country doctor of bygone years who took care of anyone (rich or poor) who fell ill in the neighborhood, crossed with a daring and sweaty guerrilla resisting his corrupt government from the distant reaches of a Latin American jungle: this chimera was the warrior-physician I secretly aspired to be.

Naively, I thought medicine was about doing the most good for the most people, through the perfect union of mind and action. Medicine was, in my exuberant and youthful imagination, more than merely an occupation; it was the highest of art forms, demanding absolute dedication to a community, with the same quiet, virtuous, and terribly passionate devotion a painter or a poet must sustain. As I grew older and read more widely, for a golden moment empathy became my dream physician's chief tool, so intangible and yet so indispensable, more incisive than his sharpest scalpel, more telling than his most advanced CT scanner. I marveled at William Carlos Williams, one of the many temporary heroes of my early adulthood, who through his poetry brought the immediacy of his particular experiences with poor patients into the consciousness of an impersonal, chaotic, and relentlessly industrializing outside American culture; for me, to become a medium for such connections was to perform the real work and drama of healing.

In the bland suburban wasteland where I grew up, I presumed snottily that most people held nondescript corporate jobs. I imagined them forced each day into gray fabric-walled cubicles, where they pushed papers across their desks and obsessed over deadlines, all in the base pursuit of maximizing profits—and the huge year-end bonuses of their companies' CEOs. My father, a highly intelligent and extremely practical man, utterly devoted to providing a decent standard of living for his family—a sometimes sad man whom I believed at times to be trapped in just such a passionless job—was patient with my self-righteousness, and from the time of my earliest memories exerted the most persistent influence on me to strive for the challenge of a career in medicine. I imagined making him proud of me, by adventurously charting the untamed and over-grown interior of the body; I would conquer the dark inner continent that might remind him of the lost Cuban home-land to which neither of us could ever return, and whose myriad wounds he had never been able to heal.

My mother, equally intelligent and hardworking but more inclined toward a vision of self-fulfillment she herself in some respects seemed to have sacrificed—an artist by training, she was the beloved (and underpaid) teacher of the learning-disabled children in the grammar school I attended—also warded me away from a career in big busi-ness, calling my attention to the imperilment of the spirit that she sensed lurked even in the spacious, walnut-pan-eled boardrooms of corporate America. She had the capac-ity to see beauty in the expressions of the body, even in the crudest of pictures her students made with clenched crayons; as both a teacher and a mother, she was my first true image of a healer. Song was her curative penicillin, language was her lifesaving bandage; poetry gave structure and definition to her classroom. While my father pushed me to take charge of my life and to become "my own boss," my mother quietly and firmly urged me to cultivate my freedom and to make proper use of the creativity she had nurtured in me.

Of course, later there were other factors that steered me toward a career in medicine, including some of the very material attractions I professed to despise. Yes, I was drawn in spite of myself to the promise of a large income, which only seemed fair recompense for the unending and grueling hours required of physicians. (So I would drive maybe an Audi or a BMW instead of a Mercedes.) Yes, I wished to join the fellowship of educated women and men, to demonstrate that I was just as capable as those in the majority culture for whom such rewarding careers seemed predestined. (So I would be passably white and straight beneath the shield of my hard-earned M.D., implicitly renouncing my queerness and my Latino origins, while taking care of those poor folk who were "less fortunate than myself" and thus "never losing sight of my roots.") Yes, yes—I would be a privileged doctor, but I would always care.

Before I had even started medical school, I found the need to brainwash myself into believing that a career in medicine still could be an instrument for social change, that it remained the noblest of callings. I concealed from myself the rich spoils signifying the profession that I began to collect everywhere, the images of success like precious silver hoarded in the bottom of a battered trunk. Like many of the epicurean Jesuit priests who taught in the Catholic high school my life partner attended, who preached to their students their version of morality and advocated a strict asceticism—while partaking of fine wines, school-funded travel to exotic locales, and sometimes the forbidden pleasures of intimacy with their young male charges—I was blind to my own hypocrisy. No price could be assigned to the restitution of health; after all, I would be taking only what the society seemed more than willing to give.

Vaguely guilty, like any good Catholic I found perverse justification in the eventual punishment for my sins, and in the long, physically exhausting, and masochistically satisfying hours spent in the hospital. Soon it became clear that the salary I was earning as a resident, considering the numbers of hours I worked, averaged in hourly pay less than the minimum wage, and so I stopped thinking about money altogether. Today, though it seems that I am assured of an emotionally challenging and intellectually satisfying job that also pays very well—general internists in the current job market, though lower paid than specialists, are in greater demand—I still do not know what medicine finally has in store for me, partly because nobody knows what society has in store for medicine. Now, as a resident working in an HMO, I am afraid to order costly tests I think my patients need, I am afraid to speak out as my residency program begins to monitor the productivity of trainees, I am afraid my anxiety may cloud my clinical judgment. I am afraid of my own bitter cynicism at the age of twenty-nine, as I stand at the threshold of a life's work that once was my most holy aspiration, as sacred an art as poetry. The more I have witnessed firsthand the inequities and the biases inherent in the current systems in place for the delivery of health care (and the more I have resorted to writing poetry as well as prescriptions), the less I have patience for the pre-approval forms for tests and utilization review decertification notices that appear in my patients' hospital charts—forms and notices through which M.B.A.'s tell me, admittedly a lowly resident, how to practice medicine. The more I put up with, the less, ultimately, I want to remain as a positive force for change in my increasingly contentious profession at all.

I once dreamed of learning how to become more empathic, not more productive; even if seduced in part by the prestige of medicine, I have never wished to be a mere cog in a new system whose sole purpose is to profit by its efficiency. Need, the oceanic depth of it, defies even the most eloquent of poems to articulate it; so how can a single telephone line to an HMO's surly triage nurse ever suffice? The monumental impassivity of the burgeoning managed–health care system, as it collides with this tidal wave of suffering, seems more likely to produce a disaster than a workable solution. Just last month, at the end of a typical clinic workweek that consisted of over sixty hours of repeated telephone calls to pharmacies to sort out which medications were covered under which HMO's formulary, filling out innumerable special TAR (Treatment Authorization Request) forms so that my MediCal patients could have access to antidepressants or the antiretroviral D4T or nicotine patches, and wrangling to get approval signatures on referral forms to allow me to send to subspecialists patients who I thought needed to be seen—not to mention the relatively small fraction of time spent in the part of my job that I actually love, which is directly caring for my patients—I attended a revelatory academic conference on the economic prospects in medicine. Though I was exhausted, at the time I was still adamant about devoting some of my time to the unreimbursed task of learning.

Like flies to a blood meal—doctors sometimes seem to love nothing more than the solemn pomp and circumstance of demise, even when it is their own collective body being picked apart—we crowded into the conference room. "Managed care" and "the future" appeared somewhere in its title, and the speaker was a faculty member in the Department of General Medicine who is a highly regarded medical ethicist and who spent most of last year not teaching at the University of California at San Francisco but instead living in hotels in Washington while working on President Clinton's task force for health care reform. He must have pictures of himself with Hillary Clinton, I thought to myself as I plunked down in a seat at the back of the room, my arms full of the charts of patients whose encounter notes from that afternoon's sessions I had yet to write. As the lights dimmed, I closed my eyes for a moment, searching the pulsing green spots that faded from my retinas for some sense of the shape of things to come, hoping to be reassured that I might still be able to accomplish something of worth as a physician of the future.

What surprised me more than anything in the talk that followed, the latest in a series of ten or so such doom-saying talks concerned with the implications of managed care, was the sense of inevitability and hopelessness in the audience as the speaker examined each traditional aspect of the modern physician's role—patient advocacy, clinical decision making, research, autonomy, benefi-cence—and not only cast into doubt its future under managed care but also questioned the a priori validity and necessity of such characteristics and functions in tomorrow's physician. The subtext to his arguments seemed to be that generalist physicians should really be no more than technicians or gatekeepers, depending upon where they were situated in the structural organiza-tion of their employer the HMO; indeed, we were no dif-ferent from (and certainly, he implicitly chastised us for our presumed self-importance, no better than) anyone else. The specialized knowledge of doctors, like that of lawyers or hotel managers or mechanics, had a price in the free-market economy and could be purchased in the same way as any other skill.

I thought for a moment of one of my demented AIDS patients, whose long-lost sense of time contrasted so glar-ingly with my own obsessive time awareness. The clinic administration, now monitoring resident productivity along with the faculty's in order to compete for large managed-care contracts, had recently cut the time allotted for patient visits from thirty to twenty minutes (a luxurious amount of time, compared to general internists attempting to provide primary care within the fifteen-minute slots given to patients in most managed-care settings). I had wished that the time we had to talk was endless, that the healing could grow to fill whatever space in time it needed, until he might remember the symptom that would tip me off to a lifesaving diagnosis. Looking around the room, I saw my disheveled and weary resident colleagues passively nodding their heads, already as defeated and confused as I in the idealistic quest to be "good doctors," too willing to berate themselves for their aspirations to what they perhaps felt in their hearts *was* a higher calling, too ready to bend themselves yet again to a demand that they were being told might ultimately benefit their patients. I felt all the more painfully the urgency in the life-defining and death-defying encounters with people brought to us by the irresistible current of illness—not simply because of the type of insurance they had or the HMO to which they belonged. The poetry that pays so little, the words that are so easily withheld, suddenly rose inside me.

Only a few years ago, I used to feel secure, at home even, in my office in the general medicine clinic where I first worked. I remember the thrill of beholding my name followed by "M.D." outside the door on my first day of seeing patients, and finding a box of business cards with that same sequence of letters (so I could not be dreaming it) tucked in a corner of the top drawer of the endearingly ugly Formica-on-metal desk in one corner of the narrow room. The chrome and goldenrod vinyl chair was an even finer example of institutional furniture, on whose armrest my elbow adhered when I tried to rise after I had listened, rapt, for a full glorious hour to the story of my first new patient. How privileged I felt to have been brought into the circle of another person's suffering, behind the heavy wooden door of my office, creating with our language our own domain of healing. The intersection of that intimacy, with the burgeoning sense of responsibility I had imposed (somewhat self-indulgently) upon myself—so great was my desire to play the knight in shining armor to my patient's two-headed dragon of disease and suffering—transformed that small office into a locus of indelible significance to me. It was a private, sheltered, possibly magical place where healing, which became merely a version of the ever-elusive mutual understanding between two individual people, could take place. No corporations, no triplicate forms, no practice guidelines interposed themselves between us. We spoke only and directly to one another.

I remember putting my stethoscope into my ears backward, later that same day when I examined another patient, and how inadequate I felt as I fumbled and apologized, only to be rescued by the knowing smile she offered me along with her knowing response—that her previous doctor, and the three before her, had also been residents at UCSF. She is still one of my most dear and devoted patients, an elderly MediCare-insured African American woman raising on her own her young grandson, who we both hope may someday become a physician himself. The pride and understanding with which she spoke erased my shame instantly, and seemed to epitomize the true mission of the physician in direct contact with a community: perhaps I only imagined it, perhaps it was part of my fantasy of what I wanted the practice of medicine to be, but I thought that when I touched her body both of us were transformed into a single new being, one that combined her wealth of experience with my willingness to learn, that matched as if in two chambers of the same heart the desire to be well and the desire to heal.

To my smallness, her great black body was the jungles of Africa and the plantations of Louisiana, laid open to me in the way only honesty of purpose can bare one person and her history to another; I was surprised that my relatively pale hands did not attempt to beat her down, but rather extended themselves toward hers as I helped her onto the examining table. When I examined her breasts for signs of malignancy, she forgave me for the countless unkindnesses of my life. When I looked at her urine under the microscope for evidence of infection, it was the most unbearable yet compelling of intimacies to which I had ever been brought. When I finally declared her free of any new diseases, I had the strange sense that I was liberating her—from the possibility that she was unclean, from the self-doubt that she was not worthy enough to be bothering a doctor, from the imagined threat of a cancerous lesion or an infection that, gone undetected, might have ended her life prematurely—or that I was in reality freeing myself from those same insidious questions about my own human worth and my own possibly defective body. In short, I identified with her, I was available to her. I was another human being simply sitting beside her, listening.

She is still alive, defying the diabetes and hypertension that threathen to make her one of the disproportionately large number of African Americans and Latinos who die of these diseases. Once she confided in me, only after quite a bit of coaxing, that she was bleeding from her vagina, an admission that led to the detection of endometrial cancer at an earlier stage than perhaps would have been possible had we never grown to trust one another enough for her to tell me about the spotting. I like to believe that in other ways I have had something to do with this "improved survival," even though she will not allow screening mammograms and refuses her yearly influenza vaccine; I like to think that empathy is instead the priceless, unbottleable, unquantifiable intervention. When I knit my brows over her elevated hemoglobin A1C, a reflection of the control of her blood sugar, she jokes with me, telling me I should not worry about her sugars getting too high, because she has always been told she was sweeter than most people, so it is in her nature to have high sugars. It is in the joking and the talking, then, and in the sharing of stories that any therapeutic influence seems to work itself out; clearly, in terms of my own well-being, it is through these human exchanges that I am constantly healing myself.

So it is all the more ironic that I must also feel guilty

when I schedule her that luxurious forty-minute slot, because it takes that long to hear about the trip she took to the country—where she picked fragrant big-as-your-hands peaches just like you get in Louisiana as their juice ran down her arms for a peach pie she baked for her grandson really which led to the slice that she should not have eaten but which was so delicious and then well that explains the high sugar reading later that day—since the practice will get reimbursed less for that time than if I saw two patients for twenty minutes each. Sometimes I feel myself confirming my own worst fears, as I scan my less productive schedule (as compared with more experienced providers who see more HMO-insured patients), where I see all the exotic names of people who need costly translators or who are late because the crosstown bus broke down: maybe she is not worth that extra expanse of time, I suppose, and maybe I am not either. Maybe neither of us can make a difference in the life of the other.

Physicians have long been remunerated by insurance companies according to how much they *do to* their patients (as opposed to how long they simply interact with them)—which, as is well known, has led to the ongoing overpopulation of subspecialty fields in which invasive procedures are performed. Since it may be impossible to assign a monetary value to such nonprocedural interactions as holding a patient's hand, I wonder how a profession that through managed care orients itself even more explicitly toward profit making and efficiency can permit space enough for this type of care. Particularly in caring for indigent patients, whose voices have already been silenced in so many other arenas, it seems barbaric to cut them off after twelve or twenty or even forty minutes have elapsed in the one place in the world where what they have to say *must* matter. When the savings (or increased earnings) that result from such reforms go toward paying huge bonuses to the presidents of HMOs and the salaries of M.B.A.'s who run these businesses, people who are answerable not primarily to their enrollees (and certainly not to patients who barely speak enough English to get their requests for appointments denied by a monolingual advice nurse) but to their stockholders, one wonders whether such changes will truly benefit the patient of the 1990s and beyond, the ill person who is more and more often referred to as the "health care consumer."

Even more alarming than the winnowing of human connections from the practice of medicine, in my view, is the decreasing power of patients in the new managed-care systems. To succeed within an HMO, individual patients must indeed become "health care consumers" more than they can allow themselves to be sick people; the most tirelessly persistent letter writers and phone callers are the ones who obtain timely access not only to providers and referrals to specialists but also to other needed services. As the primary provider of care to many people with AIDS, I have witnessed first hand how the many obstacles set in place by HMOs to obtaining care can adversely affect the health of people already struggling against a seemingly invincible disease. Asking gravely ill patients to be their own advocates (an exhausting role to which many people with AIDS are sadly already all too accustomed), while placing their physicians at a distance from them, is almost diabolical in its potential effectiveness in reducing the cost of their care.

The structure of the HMOs may make sense for the vast majority of their "clients," or at least the clients they truly compete for and do not exclude on the basis of preexisting conditions: the ostensibly healthy, happily married, young, heterosexual, not infertile couple featured recently in a television ad for one such company. Enrolling as many healthy people as possible—especially people who by the crude demographic instruments of age, marital status, ethnicity, income, and even home address can be identified as less likely to become ill—is the most penny-wise of strategies. Gay Latinos or young white women in wheelchairs or African American teenagers or homeless alcoholics do not appear in such advertisements—even if some of them may be, were, or aspire to be successful and healthy. The drawn faces of the growing number of people living courageously with AIDS will never find themselves depicted on splashy billboards along the highways of northern California—or at least not on the ones erected by HMOs. No new expensive sufferers need be encouraged to apply for benefits.

What little energies are devoted to the care of people with AIDS already enrolled in the HMO are consumed in interesting ways. A recent acrimonious conflict over delivery of care within the general medicine clinics at UCSF is a case in point. Claiming that the care provided to people

with AIDS by generalists was "too costly," without disclos-
ing the details of how this conclusion was reached (were
we ordering inappropriate tests and missing diagnoses that
led to worse, more expensive outcomes?—or spending too
much time talking to our patients, seeing them frequently
and refusing to give up on them by insisting on investigat-
ing a symptom in the hopes of uncovering a treatable condition?), one large HMO that contracts with the UCSF
clinics threatened to force all its clients with AIDS to
transfer their care to the AIDS specialty clinic. There a
small core group of specialized infectious-disease attending doctors would supervise all care through a contingent
of nurse practitioners, eliminating costly residents-in-
training. At the same time the HMO engaged the services
of a consulting group (coyly called Clinical Partners) to
police their care and to establish "reasonable guidelines"
for its delivery to people with AIDS. Clinical Partners was
to receive a certain sum of money, a smaller fraction than
the total cost of care received in the previous years for this
group of patients; any surplus above what they allowed to
be spent in caring for these people during the coming year
could be divided among themselves. Not surprisingly,
Clinical Partners sided with the HMO in the demand that
all patients with AIDS be transferred immediately to the
AIDS specialty clinic, where they thought they could
obtain the same or better care far more cheaply.

    We could not begin to gauge the potentially ill effects
of disruption of long-standing therapeutic relationships
between providers and their patients. Nor was there any

way to calculate the effects on the training of young primary care physicians (especially for an East Coast medical
school graduate like me who was advised not to waste his
precious education on a career in primary care but who
nonetheless chose to come to UCSF specifically to learn
how to provide primary care for people with AIDS), who
would be removed from any contact with this whole class
of patients. It was obvious to my patients how little regard
remained for them in the company ultimately responsible
for their care, now that the primary responsibility of their
physician, which I had always endeavored to share with
them, was indisputably being wrested from us. Worse yet,
none of us were given a voice in the decision.

Depleting invaluable reserves of spirit that should have
been channeled inward toward the struggle against this
terrifying illness, a group of residents rallied to protest
the HMO's decision. For a long time we were ignored.
Then we were told that there was no choice in the matter, an institutionalese response almost as devastating to
me as being told in medical school that AIDS was an
incurable illness. It only intensified my sense of inadequacy as a provider of care to my AIDS patients, already
a sobering and sometimes even paralyzing enemy in my
efforts to help them. In dealing with AIDS, I had long
ago relinquished any hope of control, but in this situation
I saw myself as having plainly failed my patients, the gay
men and people of color who needed me so desperately
in this battle against an impersonal system.

The decision, however, was made. Obviously, I was an

incompetent physician, a financial liability, and had previously obscured the fact beneath my dedication to caring for people with AIDS. But dedication, and even compassion, could turn out to be very costly in such an atmosphere. When one of my HIV-positive patients planned a cruise through the Caribbean, just when for the first time his T-cell count had dropped a hair below 200 on his routine every-fourth-month blood work results (placing him at the threshold for instituting trimethoprim-sulfa prophylaxis against pneumocystis pneumonia), I decided with him to postpone starting it until he returned. He had a vague history of a reaction to sulfa drugs in the past, and so I wanted to monitor him closely as he took the first few doses.

More important, as I recall, I did not want to saddle him with the burden of a new medication, an unwanted and nagging reminder of his disease, as he was about to embark on a trip so crucial and necessary to his sense of freedom and wellness. He had been planning this trip for months, his first real vacation since the death of his longtime partner from AIDS two years before, and he had shared with me demurely his hopes of possibly meeting someone new. How would it look to the other cruise ship revelers, and especially the one among them who might become his new boyfriend, if he were constantly throwing up from a new horse pill he had to down every morning? That would be the equivalent of advertising he was HIV positive, something he preferred to make known only in the context of his most intimate friendships.

So I sent him on his fabulous vacation with a smile, reassured that he would be back in only two weeks, when we would initiate the prophylactic regimen immediately. And I congratulated myself a little for having the good sense (from my sympathetic perspective as a gay man taking care of so many gay men with the disease) to allow him this one outrageous pleasure without encumbrances, to understand his desire to be alluring and sexy again without fear, to free him, if only for fourteen short days, from the worry that he might become deathly ill at any moment. As he left my office, beaming with the excitement of his imminent adventure, he promised to send me a postcard with some cute, scantily clad sailors on it. When we laughed together, again I felt that I was engaged in the process of healing. Even though we were bending ever so slightly the tiresomely explicit rules of his HMO and of its new lackeys at Clinical Partners, we had truly listened to one another and had reached our own decision.

One week later I received a complicated and distressing message. A patient of mine had called the clinic from, of all places, a cruise ship's ship-to-shore telephone, frantically trying to get in touch with me, but after several attempts had been deflected by the answering service to the physician on call for emergencies. He had suddenly become terribly short of breath and was gasping for air when he arrived at the ship's infirmary. He had a high fever, and nobody on board seemed to know what to do, including the crusty ship's doctor, who became visibly alarmed when my patient reported to him that he was HIV positive. In a growing panic, they tried to reach me during office hours but were told curtly by the telephone staff that I was busy with other patients. So they waited forty-eight hours to see whether he would improve, while he was treated presumptively for asthma. When he only continued to deteriorate, they called UCSF again, demanding to speak with someone. The physician on call for emergencies correctly diagnosed early pneumocystis pneumonia, on the basis of the classic presenting signs and symptoms, and in light of the ship doctor's lack of familiarity with AIDS, he advised urgent hospitalization. The patient, fearful that he might not receive appropriate care in the Bahamas, the next port of call on the cruise, had decided to risk flying back to San Francisco without treatment and would be arriving sometime that same evening.

Of course, I knew immediately that the patient was the man I had sent off with a pat on the back without pneumocystis prophylaxis, and that I probably would not be receiving a postcard from him after all. Though my reasoning had been well documented in the medical record, and several of my colleagues reassured me that I had done the right thing, pointing out that a week of prophylaxis probably would have done very little to prevent the infection, I still felt I had made an unforgivable mistake. Even worse, it had occurred in the glaring spotlight of the same HMO intent on proving that allowing resident physicians to care for AIDS patients was more expensive than having specialists supervise nurse practitioners. So while I worried about the state of his health, speculating as to what his oxygenation might be and trying to devise an optimal treatment strategy to employ upon his return, I found my mind partially occupied by how much more this error was going to cost the HMO. Instead of devoting my thinking entirely to his case, I was forced to consider how his illness might affect my own situation. This undesired antagonism between me and my patient, this surprising tension between my own concerns and his needs, seemed foisted upon us by a meddling, profit-hungry HMO that had no real interest in either one of us but was focused only on its own bottom line. Not only was I learning the hard way how best to manage pneumocystis pneumonia; I was also being taught the less relevant but somehow more immediately important lesson of damage control. Before the afflicted patient's airplane had even touched down, I found myself on the telephone with a clinical nurse specialist from the HMO, haggling over more expensive home intravenous pentamidine versus a cheaper trial of oral high-dose trimethoprim-sulfa, skirting the issue of why he had not been on pneumocystis prophylaxis.

Painfully absent from these events was any effort toward teaching me (as opposed to making me feel stupid) that is necessarily a part of every residency program. The training of physicians is an extremely costly process, and not only in the monetary terms cited (with little supporting data) by such groups as Clinical Partners. It has long taken place in public or veterans' hospital settings, where mostly poor people are stuck repeatedly for blood or otherwise "experimented on" (to use the sharp words of one of my own early patients who refused me a second attempt to perform a lumbar puncture). Since the transition to managed care has begun, even more of the burden of teaching medical students and residents has been shifted to the medically indigent, while the time of attending physicians in former-ly private clinic settings is more and more consumed by the exigencies of the HMO model.

So the attending physician available to consult with me on my case of pneumocystis pneumonia is in fact unavail-able when I run over to the tiny and cluttered consulting room—he is busy on the phone trying to get an echocar-diogram approved for one of his own patients, and three understandably impatient nurse practitioners are waiting for him to cosign their prescriptions. Waiting is out of the question, as even my resident's schedule is overburdened with relentless every-twenty-minutes slots. So I rush back out, doing whatever I have learned is practical but without fleshing out my limited knowledge with a discussion of the most recent data. Soon many of the best attending physi-cians will be moved out entirely, to a floor where all the HMO patients will be seen, free of the encumbrances of residents and medical students. Remaining in the residents' clinics will be all the MediCal, Medicare, and uninsured patients, creating an even more dramatically two-tiered system of health care delivery at one of the premier acad-emic medical institutions in the country.

The various barriers that my patient encountered en route to receiving, finally, his lifesaving course of IV medication—whether they were the unresponsive triage personnel manning the clinic telephones, or a distracted resident physician attempting to negotiate an openly derisive and hostile system, or the clinical nurse specialist advocating a cheaper form of therapy—demonstrate again the danger of managed competition: a greater enslavement to profit. In the same way that making money already places traditional insurers and pharmaceuticals companies at odds with all patients stricken by chronic diseases, managed-care bureaucrats who are not ultimately responsible for what happens to patients are in charge of making life-or-death decisions. Even more than the further dehumanization of medical caregiving, even more than the further burdening of the ill with the problem of self-advocacy, even more than neutralizing activism in providers of health care and limiting the education of doctors in training, it is ultimately the blatant corporatizing of health care delivery that is the most destructive element of the proposed changes to medicine. Profiting from the suffering of others is repulsive indeed.

Perhaps I am wrong, which is my greatest hope at this moment. Perhaps I am wrong, at least, about some the effects I predict the proposed changes will have upon the medical profession and the people we serve. Perhaps there is hope, even for the most depressed of residents, who wonder (as their referrals for counseling for their depressed patients are repeatedly denied) whether mental health benefits will be included in whatever plan finally is passed. Will only the already healthy—which I have long taken to mean the strong, the rich, the double-breasted suited, the very vocal, the English speaking—survive in the aftermath of this most vituperative of debates? Or can we begin, without fear, imagining the unmanaging of health care?

It Rhymes
with "Answer" ⁓

Oh what, then, did it feel like?
   I dreamed of an arrow.
And how came you to know him?
   I dreamed he was wanting.
Say the dream of him wanting.
   A swan, a wing folding.
Why do you weep now?
   I remember.
Tell what else you remember.
   The swan was mutilated.
   —Carl Phillips, from "Cortège"

Everyone has left me
except my muse,
that good nurse.
She stays in my hand,
a mild white mouse.
   —Anne Sexton, from "Flee on Your Donkey"

The lump was deeply embedded in her left breast, over her heart, whose beating I could feel transmitted through it; I discovered it with the near-lifeless tips of my left hand's fingers as I pressed down, using the steady force of only my superimposed right hand, exactly the way I had been taught over and over again in medical school and residency. The examiner's left hand should be considered merely an instrument to collect sensory information,

I recalled having been coached, perhaps so I would never recoil or gasp at the unanticipated, awful touch of a malignancy, my composure measured by my silence.

I sensed immediately, through channels unalterable by all the medical training in the world, what it was: it was tenaciously fixed against her chest wall, rock-hard in its consistency, poorly circumscribed in the breast tissue but at least three centimeters at its widest diameter. A minute, then another, passed interminably as I absorbed the consequences of the data I collected. I had just finished a month-long rotation in the breast surgery clinic at the county hospital, where I had been rushed from one examining room to another to palpate each anonymous breast just before it was to be biopsied, usually introducing myself in Spanish and hastily trying to explain to the terrified woman lying on the table in a paper gown as much of what was about to happen to her as I could, before I was ushered into yet another room. While I considered myself quite adept at recognizing the various diagnostic clinical features of breast lesions, I had no idea what comprehensible words I might say after I had found one myself that I thought was cancerous.

She was a new patient in my practice, a seventy-four-year-old Mexican woman who had been followed upstairs in the chest clinic for the last twenty years for her asthma. Every month, a physician there had listened to her heart and lungs, and yet somehow the mass had gone undetected. Apparently, nothing in particular had prompted her to consult a generalist; in the checklist review of systems, she

indicated no unusual symptoms. I spent an extra few minutes asking some direct questions, because I had encountered a disturbing number of Spanish-speaking patients
who, unable to read English and too proud to ask for help,
simply checked "no" for all the boxes on the form. She
reported that her asthma was quiescent and that she felt
generally well. All she wanted was a complete physical
examination, since she had not had one in more than ten
years. She looked oddly thin to me, the opposite of what
I expected for someone on long-term oral steroids for asthma, but she denied that she had lost weight and insisted
instead that she had been on a diet for years with unsatis-
factory results. Her husband, she remarked with a flat,
defeated voice and downcast eyes, still thought she was
too fat.

I finished as smoothly as I could the rest of her physical
exam, wondering whether in my unchoreographed pause I
had already communicated to her what I had found. Her
casually self-deprecating remark had rattled me as much as
the unwelcome presence of the lump. I myself often feared
my physical form was not satisfactory, not doctorly
enough; that, much as I wanted to strike the pose of a doctor, what people saw when they entered my office was an
ungainly imposter. My response was to focus, to discrimi-
nate, to busy myself with my mental notes. She also had
several enlarged lymph nodes in her left armpit, and a
large bruise over her right hip that she nervously said she
had not noticed, admitting only that she might have
banged her hip on a doorknob while doing the laundry. As

she dressed behind the curtain, I pondered the possibilities. Surely the cancer had spread to the lymph nodes, and
her wasted appearance suggested even more distant metas-
tases. The bruise complicated matters further: had some
renegade cells invaded her bone marrow, crowding out the
cells necessary for normal clotting, or was she a victim of
domestic violence, another life-threatening scourge of
women, and one that was vastly more common?

As I sat waiting at my desk, the tumor was taking root in
my imagination, as if my merely having detected it were
enough to assimilate it into my own body. Its anger
became my own, directed partly at a health care system
that, through a lack of Spanish-language education efforts
and an unwillingness to help shoulder the cost of care, dis-
couraged women like her from obtaining timely access to
preventive services, but also at the patient herself, for
being so passive as the disease overtook her. Given the
obviously advanced stage of her illness, I immediately
assigned her to a prognostic category that guaranteed a
miserable death. Her tumor's aberrancy mirrored me, a
physician who sometimes believed words were more curative than chemotherapy, a gay man masquerading as a professional, a Latino pretending to be competent. The blight
that I had long felt in my own chest, the gnawing dull pain
that I had often attributed to something akin to depres-
sion, assumed a more ominous shape. I was beginning to
remember, but what I felt was not yet compassion; I was
beginning to die myself, of my own occult diseases, but it
seemed more a form of suicide.

In another few moments, she was seated several feet away from me, with an expectant, slightly strained smile on her face. I said nothing. My mind had gone blank, empty of explanations, devoid of conversation, shrinking back from what it knew. When I needed most my faculties of communication, at this critical moment in the life of another human being, they failed me. I wondered whether my touch itself, instead of bespeaking comfort and human longing, had been rough and inhuman. All the familiar therapeutic mechanisms by which I knew poetry could assuage—the assignment of a name, the affirmation of identity, the propulsive translocation of metaphor, the very creation of words, and finally the possibility of authorship and control over experience—all of its power dissolved in my refusal of language. I felt as though I had finally parted company with humankind, for good. I felt myself falling, crashing downward through the momentary and terrifying failure of empathy, each layer of shared humanity like the flimsiest of cobwebs, easily broken. I was terrified not of the disease itself but of my inability to confront it with her.

It was her simple, strange gesture that saved me. Without warning, she reached out across my desk, and rested her hand lightly on my arm. My left arm. We stayed linked like that for a few minutes, communicating deeply and wordlessly. I felt the terror in her touch, and its gentleness, until it was happening to me, until I rediscovered my own narrative. I slowly smiled and began to speak effortlessly. When I told her not to be afraid, when I touched her own left arm in the spot where mine once ached, when I explained to her what she already knew was inside her, when I guided her hands to her breast to show her exactly where, what I was really telling her was a version of my own story. My own life and death, my own inconceivable cancer, was conversing with hers through the medium of our contiguous bodies; our bodies began to rhyme with one another, resonating with an experience we were on the verge of sharing. Suddenly I was in the ice-white operating room again, staring at the ceiling, absorbing the strange meaning of bad news. I was writing all my poems, over and over again, and dedicating each one of them to her. That morning, before I knew what was happening, I began to tell her my own story.

When I broke my left arm, I was skiing out of control down the steep icy face of a mountainside in upstate New York. It was only mid-October, and though the season's first snowfall was yet to come, the weather had grown cold enough to permit a full week of artificial snowmaking. The contorted, skeletal limbs of most trees were already harshly bared. The night before my fateful accident—I had awaited my first ski trip with the same brash impatience with which I entreated my eighteenth birthday, by that time less than a month away, to hurry up and come—the temperature rose so abruptly and sharply that some thought it unnatural. It climbed and climbed, by more than forty degrees and for enough hours to melt all the ski resorts' hyped-up good times in "man-made virgin conditions!" into water, only then to drop again precipitously and freeze it all into a hard sheet of ice, silvery ice that had the appearance of a huge mirror reflecting the next morning's sun as we approached. Somehow, in my teenage self-absorption and all-consuming haste, I failed to read these portents, unwilling for even a moment to attempt to contain myself, spurring myself to grow up wildly, unapologetically, recklessly.

I do remember distinctly writing a terribly maudlin poem many months later about how beautiful and particular that sunrise had seemed, how the sun had appeared to admire itself endlessly in its mountain mirror, exquisitely conscious of its ability to illuminate the world, and how at the same time it had seemed to give of itself so grudgingly to the frozen landscape and hunched-down houses that greeted its ascent. In the austere light of my traumatized memory, I re-created its rose color as reasonable and serious upon my face, and I realized in spite of myself that I was still a teenager who had allowed himself to stray a very long way from home. With a man I hardly knew. I wrote about him, too, about desiring him, about his entering me and filling my bones to bursting with a joyful music that soon became inconsolably sad. Sooner than I had expected, we had reached our destination. The dark mountain, jutting out like a silent challenge to all my nascent identities, bulging almost obscenely into my awakening consciousness, had made it clear that there would be no turning back. That was how the bad poem ended, with an implicit challenge.

Skiing was a glamorous, rich-white-kid sport that

seemed in every way contrary to my nature—Cubans in general do not understand fully the concept of snow, and tend to see only its beauty and to hear its whistling music, remaining blissfully unaware of its power to kill—but it appealed to me immensely precisely because of the various dangers it might pose. Not the least of which was the older friend who had invited me to go with him, one of the handsome waiters at the restaurant where I was running food out to the tables, a position to which I had been recently promoted from that of busboy. Now that I was more visible, not just one of the dark Mexicans who cleared his tables, he noticed me. I soon learned that he was an avid skier—and quickly grew to believe that his smile was far sexier than the high velocity he bragged about, his manner much cooler than the winter air he so relished, his body (which I had glimpsed once only briefly as we changed together into our tacky mariachi-man uniforms before the start of one of our shifts) much harder and more muscular than the sculpted mountains that gave him so much evident pleasure. He also played the guitar, the instrument of my heritage of Spanish music that I myself revered and aspired to play— even more so after watching his hands glide liquidly across the vibrating strings. I accepted his invitation without hesitation, probably too eagerly, and in doing so accepted also, and for the first time, that I was attracted to another man. Full of the adolescent's sense of his own glorious immortality and absolute invincibility, I dared to think that I could learn to ski and learn to love men simultaneously, triumphing over all the risks of getting hurt.

He picked me up before dawn, which felt terribly illicit, and I snuck out of my parents' home, leaving a brief
note on the kitchen table explaining that I had gone skiing
with a friend. I noticed the oblong arm of his guitar case
sticking up awkwardly into the back window as he pulled
up, and felt a tingle of anticipation—might he serenade me
later, in the warm arms of evening, before a roaring fire as
we relaxed after a long day on the slopes? The shared intimacies on the ride north inside his rattling blue Toyota,
beginning with the intermingling of our steamy breath and
the smoke from the several fat joints we puffed on, then
the interweaving of our words into lyrics for a song he was
writing, gave way to that spectacular view from the parking lot of the sun staring at itself and then his expert help
in clicking closed the rented ski boots and fixing them
onto the skis. Each juncture belied by its effortlessness and
joyfulness what was about to happen to me; it was as
though the cold and inhospitable world, despite what I
had been taught about how it could punish the rule break-
ers, were going to allow my life to happen. My very future
seemed to be opening up to new possibilities as we rose
side by side on the ski lift beyond the level of the treetops,
until we nearly reached the thin clouds that swirled fanci-
fully in the blue sky at the rocky peak's pinnacle.

Before I knew it, we were released onto the bright white
trail. Exhilaration became wings upon my shoulders. The
feeling re-created in my mind that of the meeting of a
sharpened pencil and a blank sheet of the whitest paper.
The accident seemed to occur just as I was achieving

flight, the rush of the cold air past my ears and across my face identical to the feeling of adrenaline needling through my body, just as I was approaching a climax—I had never been so high in my entire brief life, a conspiracy of the great altitude and the powerful marijuana. Gravity, acceleration, force, inertia—all the data my senses collected— each was reinterpreted by my brain, and my calculations told me that I was capable of take off, my skis hissing their agreement as I picked up speed, my new buddy only split seconds ahead of me. What I had only dreamed about in poetry, what I had only fantasized about alone in bed, was suddenly about to occur. I braced myself for the ecstasy of catching up to him and then being locked arm in muscled arm, naked as the lightening sky, rising farther and farther above the unforgiving world, in amazing and impossibly musical flight.

The soft internal sound of the bone breaking was akin to not hearing the whispering of some unspeakably important secret; the intense pain I felt caused me to cry out dumbly, as though I had been given the secret of eternal life and for a fleeting moment actually understood it. I was slipping, I was in the process of being betrayed. The earth wanted me back, and reclaimed me brutally as I skidded face-first down the hill, so brutally that I thought I had left vital parts of myself strewn behind me in my wake. I learned that the price for flight, no matter how brief that period of flight might be, was to be pressed face to chest to thigh to toe against the ground, to be eternally weighed down by the body itself. What I could see now of the rest of my life consisted of one loose ski clattering aimlessly away from me, downward, downward, farther and farther into the imminent and inescapable blackness. The man I had barely loved, and at so great a cost—I was certain I would die then, before I ever even imagined the existence of AIDS, before my grandfather renounced Cuba on his deathbed, before I published my first poem, before I came out as a gay man to my family, before I helped to split open the chest of a victim of a gunshot wound or diagnosed cancer or administered a course of toxic chemotherapy—the man who led me down the path of such promise and its inevitable destruction, the man who caused the future and not my past to flash before my stunned eyes, had disappeared into the distance. And I never saw him again.

The ski patrol saved me from the most obvious ways I might have died, bundling me in warm blankets like the most fragile and precious of packages before placing me gingerly in the yellow banana sled that they used to transport accident victims to safety. Anything inside me might break or be broken, and I saw the possibilities in their eyes. Had I been unconscious for minutes or hours, or only a few seconds? I thought I was bleeding, I suspected that something precious was seeping out of my body, but I did not know from where. Instinctively I looked for the sun up in the sky, but I lacked the survival skills to divine by its position what time of day it might be; I was so shocked, I was barely capable of feeling its weak warmth on my face. The members of the ski patrol looked upon me not with pity but with an urgency that seemed to express both kindness and revulsion. I was an emergency to them, a person in need, a task, a logistical problem, the reason they had chosen this work. When one of them smiled at me and handed me his woolen hat—I had lost mine, which seemed emblematic of my confused mental state, somewhere above us—I knew from staring at his bared teeth that something terrible was happening to me and that perhaps I was not really being saved. Another of them then fashioned a clumsy cravat from a piece of cloth, and before I could protest, not really convinced that I wanted to go on living, we were zigzagging down the hill, the group of them far enough ahead to give me the impression that they were toying with the idea of abandoning me to a fate I somehow deserved, but could not in the end bring themselves to do it.

All my impatience, all my self-destructiveness, all my awkward poetic utterances, all my arguments with my parents seemed somehow to be concentrated in the screaming now emanating from my left arm. The acceleration of my growing up, which I so desperately yearned for in my speeding down the hill, was now converted into whatever was happening in this dangling extremity of mine. The propensity for uncontrolled growth was inside of me, and I knew it; just as I had acknowledged my queerness, that most insatiable of appetites that led (as I had been taught) the men whom it afflicted to a self-consuming number of sexual partners, my physical body was already revealing its own ability to consume itself. But I was not capable of making these interpretations at the time. Instead, I fixed my eyes only upon the red crosses fluttering on white flags in the distance at the bottom of the hill, promising me shelter and a kind of safety.

The first doctor I saw was a well-tanned and wind-burned orthopedic surgeon, who probably worked in the ski patrol's emergency tent once each season in exchange for free lift tickets. He smiled and rolled his eyes as he picked a few pine needles out of my hair—which reminded me not only of how my descent had been so jarringly halted but also of how childish and dependent I must have appeared to him—before proceeding to ask me several blunt questions and then announcing with a half yawn that he thought my arm might be broken. Apparently, he had seen more than his fair share of stoned seventeen-year-old novice skiers with broken arms. Then he handed me a mimeographed page of complicated directions to the nearest hospital—"It's only about a twenty-minute drive, and the splint I'm putting on should hold you together until you get there. Didn't you come with some friends or something?"—and sent me on my way without even examining me more closely, partly because for some reason we could not peel my jacket off the injured arm and I refused to let him cut to pieces my snazzy new two-hundred-dollar advance birthday present. Too ashamed to admit I had been deserted, in excruciating pain despite the blunting effect of the marijuana I had smoked still circulating in my system, I stumbled out of the tent in my rigid rented ski boots, dazed and with my useless arm pressed close against my chest in my new sling. The few tears I shed froze bitterly in my eyelashes, and my left hand (which even then, it seemed to me, in light of its newly imposed intimacy with the rest of my bruised body—or alternatively, in its oddly enforced new gesture of unwavering devotion—I had never trusted) grew ever more sinister looking as it began to turn from pink to dusky blue in color. It then dawned on me, as my arm seemed to take on this strange personality of its own: why had I broken it after my very first and relatively trivial wipeout?

I had always secretly suspected that I might be physically defective, that I might have soft bones or hidden deformities that were a consequence, or maybe the root of, or perhaps some kind of physical echo of what I considered to be my various character flaws. I had long feared that something internal might break whenever I wrote, because I seemed to press down too hard with my pen, it seemed too important to me that I do it well. Another self-punishment that masqueraded as a fear that day: perhaps I would never write again at all. My outward, dramatic pose of immortality was merely a façade, an antidote to my low self-esteem. In this regard I was no different from most teenagers. But I was different in other ways, and it was becoming harder and harder to deny my "weirdness." As I spotted a group of my younger brother's druggie friends farther down the hill, punching each other in the exact place my arm seemed to have been broken, laughing and calling each other "faggot" and "pussy" with an absolute confidence that it could never be so, that no male friend in their group could ever be queer, I felt my alienation all the more keenly. Pathetic and demoralized, with no other recourse, I approached them feebly to ask for help. My arm was throbbing more insistently, desiring attention now with an almost sexual intensity.

Miraculously, one of them offered me a ride to the hospital without the attendant humiliation and derision I had anticipated. No jokes about who might have ditched me, no rolled eyes or uncontrolled spasmodic giggles. My arm seemed to inspire pity and consternation in even the most potentially unsympathetic people—like the orthopedic surgeon pulling the pine needles from my long hair—as though its own inherent softness could be transmitted to the hearts of others. But by then my perceptions were beginning to fade, and I recall feeling quite dizzy, and as though my life were unraveling, as we spiraled down the mountain road toward the hospital. By the time we arrived at the emergency room, I was semiconscious and only barely able to give my name and my parents' phone number to the triage nurse who greeted us and then ushered me inside. This time, when huge metal shears appeared from a drawer to cut off the tense sleeve of my new ski jacket that covered my injured arm—it had swollen by that time to the size of my thigh—I was unable to resist. I was not prepared for what I saw underneath. The sight of my own black-red blood saturating the goose-down filling of the sleeve, and then the jagged, beak-like projection of the white and red-speckled bone piercing through the skin caused me to lose consciousness. The ink of my blood, the sharp quill of my bone—a terrible poem as yet unwritten, but soon to take shape. When I came to a few moments later, it was to the concerned face of the nurse saying that I was going to get a shot of Demerol and Valium, that the medicine would burn a little but would help me sleep while they reset the bone.

The next time I awoke, I was in a hospital bed and it was dark. I was alone in the oversized room, and a meal tray with domed plate covers loomed like a miniature mountain range beside me, on my left. On my left, on my left, the scene of my unmaking—then I remembered my grotesque arm, which jolted me with a burst of electrical pain when I tried reflexively to move it. I discovered that it was encased again, protected and hidden from my sight, but now more definitively in a rock-hard, ghostly white cast. A glowing clock, which I mistook at first for the moon, loomed above me, and I stared at it skeptically as an endless minute passed. The prospect of my own mortality was all around me, and even though I kept telling myself it was only a bro-ken bone, likely to require merely an overnight stay before I went home with some pain pills, the eerie solitude and humming quiet of the hospital late at night suggested to me that my prognosis might in fact be much more grave. I noticed the gaping door to my room, oversized to allow for the passage of patients in gurneys, but my imagination turned it into a portal for departing souls too expansive to fit through human-sized openings. All night, intermittent-ly delirious from the pain medication I had received, I tor-tured myself with morbid thoughts, conjuring an evil grin in the gleaming metal sink in one corner of the room, imagining the night that washed over me through the huge windows to be an infinite black river of death.

The next morning my pinched-faced parents retrieved me, and their scolding in the car on the way home restored to me my sense of vitality—I argued contemptuously with them about my decision to go skiing without their permission, and their confessions of a sleepless, worried night waiting up for me when I did not come home only fortified me more. Several weeks later, at a loss to explain the continued paralysis of my left hand, my regular doctor referred us to a world-renowned orthopedic surgeon at Columbia. In a matter of those few weeks, my wounded arm had become less a source of terror or a reminder of my weakness than a badge of my independence. It had been reconfigured almost immediately into a status symbol when I had returned to school. It grew colorful with the Magic Marker inscriptions of my friends, as colorful as the exaggerated and glamorized version of the story of the accident with which I regaled them as they scribbled their get-well messages. It was cool to have been injured while defying the overprotective and restrictive world that surrounded us, where even the physical force of gravity seemed to be on "their side." So when this gray-haired expert told us that he thought the radial nerve, one of the large and important nerves that ran along my fractured humerus, was damaged, maybe permanently, I was almost overjoyed, much as I disbelieved him. I was sure my arm would function normally again, that this old fart did not have the power to make any pronouncement on the state of my health, but until then I would enjoy the novelty of being paralyzed. I could hardly wait to horrify my new-found friends with the unfortunate news.

When the cast finally came off a few weeks later, however, the interest in my bravado and tale-telling had long since faded. Beneath the cast, atrophied and pale and sour smelling, was my defective arm. A small irregular scar had formed where the broken bone had punctured the skin, and my wrist drooped down like a swishy hairdresser's when the support of the plaster was withdrawn. I was surprised by how heavy my left hand seemed, as though I could feel in it for the first time the weight of all its accumulated and unappreciated tasks—after all, though I was technically ambidextrous, I always preferred to use my right hand. Now I tried solicitously to extend my scorned left hand, gracefully to bend it back, but the useless thing only flopped downward, obeying gravity instead. I realized as the skin was stretched over the back of my wrist that it was numb, in a triangular patch at the base of my thumb, as though an invisibly tattooed message had been inscribed there by a sage and the anesthetic had not yet worn off. Though there was no pain, and nothing I could think to do with my left hand at the moment, still I felt the tears well up in my eyes.

The wrist drop with which I lived over the next several months was like having my queerness branded physically upon me. All my efforts to conceal my sexuality seemed thwarted by this constant reminder of my acquiescence to that unhealthiest of impulses. What was most incredible to me was that merely the acknowledgment of an attraction was enough to have marked my physical body—that I was being punished without even ever having committed the sin. Though I was given a blue plastic-and-Velcro brace, which maintained the wrist in a neutral position, I felt an odd and self-punitive compulsion to remove the brace before my friends and demonstrate my disability. On some level, I wanted them to know, wanted them to understand how it was a part of me. Whatever sympathy or admiration they felt for me had vanished, however—now I was nothing more than a circus sideshow, like the hermaphrodite or the bearded lady. Indeed, I was diseased not only in terms of my exposed homosexuality but also in a more readily understandable way: the first time I heard the word "cancer" used in connection with my arm was when one of the girls before whom I performed, shaking my wrist limply like a dead small animal, shrieked out at me to get away from her—how could I be sure that I didn't have it? What if I had *cancer*?

What if the faggot had cancer? And if I did, was it contagious in the way that homosexuality or tropical diseases were considered to be? The thought had never fully entered my mind. Even when I had been shown the ominously shadowy X ray, into which I had peered as if into the darkest of dungeons, and the orthopedic surgeon pointed out to me what he described as a benign bone cyst that had been the underlying cause of the fracture, the possibility of cancer had been so terrifying that I had simply repressed it. My parents would not ask the question;

the specialists would not mention it. We all wanted not to believe the worst—and why should we?—all indications were that this cyst was benign. Then, suddenly and cruelly as the tumor itself, there it was, jaws gaping wide: the word had been said. She could not have more accurate, connecting as she did my most barely hidden pathologies. And everything began to make sense. Yes, it might require surgical intervention, something might have to be cut off. The hungry, genetically abnormal cells that nobody believed were lurking in my arm began slowly to eat their way through my defenses.

Years later, two weeks before I was due to graduate from Harvard Medical School, I took a pile of my old X rays to one of the most famous of the world's bone oncologists. The man I loved, and who loved me, had cajoled me into doing it. I was having some pain in my arm, very minor, hardly worth mentioning. After all, I was about to graduate from one of the world's great medical schools, so how could anything possibly be wrong with me? Had I not written poetry, therapeutic poetry, the words transmitted across the long-dormant, presumptively benign lesion, then through my toothy old typewriter, onto the forgiving page? Had I not finally exorcised from myself the cruelty of the Catholic Church, which taught me that my love was evil? Those early poems, full of the kind of self-conscious music one sings to oneself to ward off demons, a kind of nervous whistling through the dark woods of my late adolescence, gave no real clues as to the true nature of what I might contain. In the process of becoming an adult, I had reassured myself over and over again that I had been cured of all my old superstitions—-that in my scarred arm might be hidden a punishment for my homosexuality or an undecipherable map of my unexplored Cuban rain forests, that bad people got bad diseases, that I might have an undiagnosed cancer. An operation before I left home for Amherst College had restored most of the function to my injured radial nerve, follow-up physical therapy had built back up most of my arm's strength, and serial X rays had revealed no change in the bone cyst—which was only the tiniest bit disconcerting, since I was told that such cysts were commonly stimulated to heal by the regrowth of bone across any resultant fractures. While I had been advised to continue with the periodic X rays, when it became clear after the first two or three years that no changes in the cyst had occurred, I simply stopped going. I was afraid of subjecting myself to repeated doses of radiation, more than I was afraid of what it might be able to find in me. At least that was how I rationalized my behavior.

I wanted to say what it was now. Out loud. After all, "cancer" is only a word, like any other. After the appointment was over and I had listened calmly to it as it was said to me, after I heard this famous doctor say matter-of-factly that he thought I might have cancer, I practiced saying it myself over and over again. I was rehearsing on the stage of my own mortality once again, but this time the performance seemed inevitable. The word reverberated in the absolute silence that my mind's audience had instantly become; I gripped it in my mind's fist like a hot stone, unable to throw it far from me, letting it burn into my skin. I was angry, I wanted to hit people with it. Then, the next moment I wanted to make a prayer out of it, I wanted to write a poem with it. It is a beautiful word, forceful and piercing, and I wanted desperately to own it in a cognitive or verbal way, because to do so might help neutralize whatever it was doing to me that was beyond my control. For the first time, I began to understand what my patients meant when they said they were visualizing their tumors shrinking, or imagining their body's natural defenses killing individual tumor cells, because my immediate impulse to write about my own cancer was one of enclosure, of limiting, of self-control. I wanted to build walls of words around it, I wanted to make its unregulated, mutant, renegade cells conform to my order and structure. I wanted to suffuse it in sonnets, I wanted to love it into remission. It became clear to me that my body's natural defenses, if I possessed any at all, were the sounds and rhythms of my own persisting physical body, a music that could not be squelched. And so I made myself a mental note: that "cancer" rhymed with "answer." When I got home, I cried in the bathroom for three hours.

Ironically, anything I may have learned in medical school that might have helped me combat this disease seemed ineffectual and irrelevant. It was to poetry that I instinctively and immediately turned, to the healing words of Audre Lorde and later to those of Sonny Wainwright, and not to the one-thousand-page oncology textbook recommended by my professors. Perhaps I had seen too many patients die miserably of their cancers, even as the next dose of some hideously orange-colored, last-resort chemotherapy they were receiving was infused into their veins to the impartial hum of IV pumps. Perhaps what I had seen—in medicine the old taboos and silences about cancer seemed always to dominate the response to people living with the disease—propelled me toward another realm of healing. Even as I was being informed of my own likely diagnosis, I felt the door to that posh, tastefully decorated doctor's office gradually closing, I imagined my stammering, ungraceful questions being stymied. I felt a possibly unquenchable thirst for words, the music of language that might comfort me in the hour of my own greatest need, to take the place of the hands of the Catholic priest who would not be ministering to the last rites. Poetry would be my desperate trip to Mexico for Laetrile, my tolerant and accepting religion, my blood-curdling battle cry and my invective, my dream of a cancer-free future.

However, many challenges to what might be called my passionate faith in the healing powers of poetry were to come before it reached its fullest realization in me. The first test I underwent was a CT scan, which was needed to delineate more clearly the appearance of the abnormal bone. Depending on what it showed, I might go home with either a great sense of relief or a next-day appointment for a biopsy. As I entered the humming machine under the bone oncologist's order, the console became a futuristic altar before which I was to be sacrificed. I tried for the last time to discern the mysterious working of the

Lord in whom my parents had taught me to believe, mes-
merized by the scanner's blinking readouts and praying
desperately beneath the cool white sheet of fluorescent
light for my salvation, but the red digital numbers seemed
instead simply to be cataloging each of my transgressions
in an undecipherable code. I imagined I felt the X rays
penetrating my tissues as the images were made, like the
fingers of a higher being touching the bone itself, but its
touch was neither healing (as I wished it would be) nor
absolving—it was quite unconscious, merely an instrument
gathering its data coolly and dispassionately. I should have
known I was alone from the moment when the bespectacled technician stepped behind his thick leaded partition
before calling out to me the command "Don't breathe!"

Since the last time I was in a scanner (as a child for the
evaluation of severe headaches that turned out to be "psychological"), I had learned a great deal, too much, in fact,
so even the possible magical properties of the device were
no longer available to me. Therefore I concentrated on
trying to remain savvy, or at least to feel that way, as precise and unerring as an X ray beam, thinking in the
absence of a God that would save me that I must save
myself. Technology was the master of my fate, in the
world of modern medicine in which I had been trained,
where an MRI was worth a thousand words. My own
interactions with patients, which until that time had consisted primarily of subjecting them to tests like this one,
returned to me as the scanner hummed and whirred.
Instead of sitting down at their bedsides to hear the sto-

ries I knew they contained, I had tried to tell them what the results of the tests meant. Instead of listening to their plans for the trip to the Caribbean they had been meaning to make, I had tried to make them understand their prognoses. I had tried to be strong, extending my robot-like arms to pull them onto the gurneys that would take them to their radiation treatments, but I had never embraced them. Always, because it was my job, I tried to know more than I felt.

When the CT scan confirmed my bone oncologist's suspicions, a biopsy of the abnormal area was scheduled for the next day. Again, I tried to steel myself, this time into the sharpest of needles, like the one that would penetrate the cortex of my humerus in search of a definitive tissue diagnosis. All that night I read the textbooks I had initially spurned, forsaking my journal and its poetic ruminations, honing my knowledge into a blade, something that could cut through all the overlying soft layers of helplessness and reassurance and hope, to get through to the undeniable truth. I divided the muscles that stood in my path and, in doing so, attempted to understand weakness and strength from a purely anatomical perspective. There was still the chance that this lesion was benign, something like fibrous dysplasia or an osteoid osteoma. Alternative diagnoses rose and populated my yearning imagination. But my efforts, in the end, were to no avail; as the night wore on, my arm grew more and more disconnected from my body. I was in the process of disowning it, in spite of my desire to understand it, preparing myself for the possibility that I would awaken in the afternoon the next day disconnected from it, utterly without it.

So I consciously made my left arm the repository of all that I had so long loathed about myself. My queerness again inhabited this part of my body, as it had when my wrist drooped so effeminately. The shameful, tentative poetry I wrote, itself a signifier of my homosexuality, I also banished to this forbidden zone, and its ungainliness I excused on the basis of faulty hard-wiring that was beyond my control. Even Cuba, cut off from the United States politically and economically since around the time of my birth, seemed to reside more in that tangled jungle of wildly overgrown cells than in any other place in my body; the pain I felt was a kind of internal equatorial heat rising up from that spot. My dismemberment would serve a purpose after all, a ritual by which I might rid myself of all that I detested, or all that was detestable in me to others. After all, my bone oncologist had been blunt: If they found what looked grossly to be cancerous and if it was too extensive to be debrided, they might be forced to amputate right then and there, and I had to give my consent in advance. I did so, almost gratefully.

I then imagined myself as the strangely asymmetric being I might become. I was not a candidate for rebuilding—I was hardly even American, and not even a close approximation of television's patriotic, heterosexual, and white Six Million Dollar Man. The U.S. government would sooner spend that amount of money in an effort to deport me, in order to avoid providing me with any dis-

ability benefits. I tried on various other personae, both ani-
mate and inanimate: the unlucky and fast-living one-armed
bandit of the slot machine emptying itself of coins, the
veteran-hero of a meaningless war who begged for money
on a city street corner, the ruined armless statue that could
still teach about beauty, the broken-winged bird I once
found flopping about trying to fly out from beneath the
front window of my parents' house. I thought maybe I
could be happy; I thought of my parents videotaping me
waterskiing or rock climbing with one arm. I thought I
might become proof of the amazing, a symbol of the anything that someone is always saying is possible. I wondered whether I would walk differently, losing my innate
sense of balance. To complete my new identity, I even
imagined prevailing against a faceless intruder into my
future home who would run off screaming when my pros-
thetic arm was torn off during our scuffle. As I slept that
night, these were my distorted dreams, my nightmares of
self-mutilation.

Perhaps more painful and disturbing than even the
remote possibility of losing my arm was a discussion I had
with one of the orthopedic residents during my preoperative evaluation early the next morning. Included in the
routine questionnaire was a series of questions clearly
designed to assess risk of exposure to the AIDS virus. *Circle
any that apply: homosexual, intravenous drug user, past blood prod-
ucts/transfusions recipient.* I knew my risk of infection through
sex was nonexistent, since I had been in a mutually
monogamous relationship with the same man for the past

seven years, and both of us had tested negative for antibodies to HIV at the start of our relationship, and had
remained so more than six months later when we were
retested before enrolling in medical school. I considered
my occupation as a medical student to be far more risky
than my sex life with regard to the possibility of HIV
exposure. Gradually, I felt my rage begin to burn in my
face and my ears. What difference did a patient's HIV risk
factors make to them, surgeons who should be using the
well-documented "universal precautions" that had been
adopted during the height of the AIDS epidemic? If I circled the word "homosexual"—the label itself was enough
to put you at high risk, apparently, without regard to number of partners or even sexual practices—would they
refuse to operate on me unless I agreed to an HIV test, like
the notorious orthopedist at Stanford University who had
been in the news for her stand on this issue? Or would
they simply test me without my informed consent, secretly sending an extra tube of blood down to the laboratory
as I had seen done on at least two separate occasions during my surgery rotation at another Harvard hospital?
Having witnessed silently what some gay patients had
been subjected to, from outright hostility to relative
neglect to behind-their-backs jokes, I decided to remain
silent on this questionnaire, too. I wrote in "medical student" and circled it. If I had to warn them of something, I
considered myself guilty only of that.

The resident, a young, anemic-looking blond man
whose gold wedding band made it clear he had achieved

the social milestone of marriage, glanced wearily over my answers. I knew how he felt, guessing by his heavy eyelids and disheveled hair that he had been up most of the previous night. He frowned and then asked me what I meant by writing in and circling "medical student." I replied by saying that I thought being a medical student put me at some risk for HIV exposure. His suspicions thus aroused, he asked me whether I had ever been tested, and I lied and said no. He scribbled something on the questionnaire and then looked more closely at me, squinting, as though he might be able to tell by my appearance whether I was indeed virus free. His eyes darted quickly to my left ring finger, where the diamond-and-sapphire ring my partner had given me as a symbol of our own private commitment to one another—no ceremony required—sparkled in the antiseptic light. He then commented on it, quite coolly, as if he had just happened to notice it, complimenting my wife's taste and adding how interesting it was to see another nontraditional wedding band; more and more people seemed to be getting creative with them. After several awkward seconds passed, during which again I held my tongue, he smiled almost smugly, perhaps sensing his victory. To this day, I wonder whether in an effort to protect himself he tested me for AIDS without my knowledge, whenever I picture his gloved hands drawing that single extra tube of blood from my vein—"just in case one of the others gets broken or lost."

Of all the silences and unspoken words across which I had groped for understanding during the evolution of my illness, it was this one that finally overwhelmed my defenses. Could they really refuse me the biopsy procedure if they had tested me and I was positive? The implicit threat that I might not even get my diagnosis infuriated me—and if I had cancer, then the potentially curative surgery I needed urgently would be indefinitely delayed by my not knowing the diagnosis. When I returned home this time, I headed directly for my desk and swept aside all those textbooks with one wide swoop of my arm—my left arm. I hoisted my typewriter into the cleared space and began to write. The poems poured forth from me like a swollen river after a storm, and through them I relived the pain of my original accident, and then I took myself through the horrible amputation, through the courses of toxic chemotherapy, through my eventual abandonment by my family and loved ones, all the way through to my death. I was writing sonnets, love poems, like the ones I long before had imagined, and the words were spilling from my brain down into my chest and filling my arms, both arms, and finally moving into my hands and fingers so they could be typed onto the page. I could barely keep up with them, and with each fresh sheet of paper I felt as though I were passing through it into another realm, as though my very consciousness were being passed through one clean white filter after another, until all that was left was light, a pure white light that penetrated and illuminated me more powerfully than any X ray.

When I finally rested, thirty-two sonnets were piled to the left of the typewriter and I was breathing rapidly. My heart was pounding so urgently it was like a fist on a table. My fingertips tingled where they had struck the lettered keys over and over again. I had a terrifically fat hard-on. I was filled with a sense of my own well-being; I felt restored to health. I had discovered through these poems what awaited me after death—it was unknowable, indeed, but it also had a great and fantastic musical language. It could be spoken, but only with the realization that after death the body's organs were all rearranged, like one's boxed possessions after a move to a distant country: heart became mouth, eyes became tongue, ears became lungs. "Arm" half rhymed with "song" and "cancer" uncannily with "answer." In my sudden seizure of need to find my own cure, I had found poetry right where I had left it. It was deep in my bones all along, in the marrow, in my long bones that dreamed of being made into flutes whenever I did die, even in my smallest bones that might someday be another man's trinkets. But at that revelatory moment, they were all still singing with life, singing that it was not yet my time.

The next day, when the anesthesia carried me away while the surgery was performed, I left consciousness knowing I would return to it intact. I knew my arm was healing itself, knew that whatever transformations its constituent cells had undergone, they were now nonmalignant. The biopsy in fact ultimately revealed fibrous dysplasia, which explained my symptoms of pain and the abnormal appearance of the bone on X ray. The surgeons removed as much of the dysplastic tissue as was possible— I was reminded somberly after it was all over that fibrous dysplasia may be a precancerous condition—and they packed the resultant cavity with normal bone taken from an anonymous donor's hip. Such a sharing it is to contain a part of another person, to have such a peculiar and unrepayable gift, from one body directly to another, just as the heart gives itself to the poem on the page, all without the possibility of the recipient's even expressing his gratitude. What another gave, and what I gave myself, is all that I needed to survive.

So it was with my patient, who we together did discover had advanced breast cancer—the biopsy was performed the next day, after a mammogram confirmed the exact location of the mass, which looked on the film like a large white moth trapped in tar. Though she was unluckier than I had been, with the cancer, as I had suspected, already metastatic to her lymph nodes and liver, I believe that she nonetheless found a kind of healing in guiding me through my own memories of a brush with death. What she gave me, and what I hoped I gave her, was a place to begin, a means by which to comprehend. I was amazed when she brought me poems of her own one day, poems that gave her lost breast a name, poems that got her through the chemotherapy because she always told herself she had so much more to write. The inner resources I believed prejudiciously she might lack on that fateful morning of our first meeting instead turned out to be prodigious, enough to sustain us both. Her last six months on this earth, I believe, could have been possible only through the astonishing record of them that she left behind.

Sometimes, when I let my thoughts roam aimlessly through my body, they investigate the traumatized area of my arm; I returned there again when my patient with breast cancer touched me where I was healed. She hardly winced as she read the poems in my eyes, in the shape of the bone, in the tears that trickled down my face as I remembered. With her looking on, now from her far-off vantage point, I wonder at what may have happened here, what still might happen. Like a blinking tourist inspecting a strange rock formation in the desert, one that is as inhospitable as it is curiously attractive, when the stinging wind of anger blows, I leave in search of another, more welcoming place. Sometimes, when the wind blows more gently, I imagine I hear beautiful music.

Giving It Back ⁓

Musing over my future career options as a physician, the dean of student affairs at Harvard Medical School mentioned something about my "giving back to the community." Puzzled by what she meant, I wondered what it was that I could have unwittingly stolen. (Having grown up in white America, I suppose I must have been taught that the dark one in the room must always be guilty of *something;* in my case especially, this was usually in fact true.) It seemed virtually impossible to me that I owed anybody anything, given the history of numbing loss that was all that I had inherited from my Cuban relatives. Indeed, it seemed to me that someday reparations would have to be made to *me*, for the lost sugar plantation and the one thousand slaughtered head of cattle, for the nameless stream that ran with our blood and the salt and sand quarries in which our murdered bodies were dumped—all that was my birthright as proved by the yellowing deed I imagined my grandfather clenching in his fist as he tearfully told and retold his stories of the revolution.

So what could I now give back, one who had so very little, one who was still so busy trying to make his selections? Yes, the Americans had turned their backs on us at a crucial moment, but in the end they had given us a new home in a glaring white supermarket of opportunities, bargains, and possibilities. The point of my American journey seemed to be what else I could acquire, the state-of-the-art home entertainment center or the the swank beachfront vacation home in Florida, each more clearly imaginable to me than my grandfather's out-of-tune guitar or the modest house that faced toward the sea from which he and his family had once made their dramatic escape. As I listened impatiently to the dean wax eloquent on the needs of poor Latinos (who lived in neighborhoods through which I would avoid driving if at all possible, people who might try to pay me for my services with chickens or tortillas, people whose teenage sons I worried might mug me on my way home from a night shift in the emergency room), I grew more and more concerned about paying back the sixty thousand dollars in student loans I had amassed during my academic career. I was contemplating a lucrative

career in diagnostic radiology—whatever youthful idealism I had brought with me to medicine had long since
evaporated. I had started to like the fluid look of my reflection in the shiny Volvos and BMWs parked around the
hospital in the spaces reserved for the radiologists as I
walked in each day; I liked having my boundaries blurred.
What could be wrong with the soft, pink, perfectly made
body of success? I wanted to wear America like an expensive suit, the best that money could buy. I deserved it.

Of course, I conceded on some level that there were others like me who had been dispossessed as well, perhaps just
as unfairly, those same Spanish-speaking people from so
many cultures, races, and nations who were fast becoming
my patients as I embarked on my first ward rotations. I saw
too how what they had lost oftentimes was recorded physically upon their bodies: the missing limb, amputated after
an inadvertent step on a land mine, the empty eye socket,
where the globe had been ruptured after a gun butt's brutal
blow to the face, the lost uterus, removed during an aggres-
sively promoted government sterilization program.
Sometimes their illnesses were less obviously caused by the
conditions in which they were now forced to live, or the
jobs hunger urged them to take: the green-eyed woman
from Mexico who burned her arm in the hungry maw of a
laundry press, the gray-haired Salvadoran man with scarred
lungs and a nerve disorder who probably had inhaled pes-
ticides sprayed while he was picking fruit, the cinnamon-
black man from Cuba whose infant daughter was bitten by
a hungry rat in the housing projects where they lived. I felt

sorry for them, to be sure, but if there was one thing I had by then learned during medical school it was how to protect (if not exactly to take care of) myself.

Moreover, my own once downtrodden family of immigrants had not only survived but prospered. Despite their own personal litany of hardships—the omnipresent language barrier, the matter-of-fact but subtle discrimination, and the especially savored moments of blatant persecution—their durability, much more than their industrious achievements, had been always a source of great pride to them. So I expected no less of these people for whom I was beginning to care, whose bodies were my laboratories and my classrooms. If they were vaguely "my people," it was more in the sense of "property" or "baggage" as opposed to "spirit." The myth of the uniqueness of fingerprints was making a dangerous kind of sense to me; human beings were so inalterably different, even when they shared a dietary staple or a mother tongue or an unsurprising susceptibility to bullets, that I believed it was impossible for an embrace or a prayer or a handshake or even a poem to bring them together.

Then there was the larger problem of what was meant by "community" in the first place. Was this well-intentioned dean referring, when she pronounced this polysyllabic word, only to the Cuban expatriate community, whose rabid patriotism and reactionary anticommunist/anti-Castro right-wing politics repulsed me, but to whom I nonetheless belonged in the most obvious ways? Or did she mean the more broadly defined Latino community, which in Boston at the time comprised not only Cubans but also much larger contingents of Dominicans and Salvadorans, as well as a significant number of Puerto Ricans (some born on the U.S. mainland, some back on the island itself) and a growing number of Mexican Americans? Or, perhaps worst of all, did she simply relegate me to the most broadly defined category available, that clamoring undifferentiated heap of the darker-skinned oppressed, those pitiably disadvantaged and generically "poor" people in America? Or were there other groups of people—ones I was afraid to acknowledge in her genteel presence, or even others at the moment unknown to both of us—with whom I shared yet another different homeland?

I had felt many times, or been made to feel, that I had been admitted to Harvard Medical School for a very specific reason. I was not really expected to think independently or to have original ideas, but to satisfy a quota, to represent someone's stereotype of the Latino student—who, by definition, could not aspire to a career in research or in some high-powered superspecialty but instead, after his brief elevation into the world of privilege, would dutifully go back out into his underserved "community" to practice medicine. Less intellectually demanding jobs existed for me in the ghettos; there were always plenty of openings there for relatively low-paid primary care providers. Disenfranchised as I was often presumed to be, I was forced to play that most thankless of roles, that of the one who desperately needs that life-changing hand up. Presumably, otherwise I might have made nothing of

myself. This particular recasting of my identity was especially painful to bear, because it was authored by the acts
and attitudes of the kindly liberal people who I knew were
allies, people who wanted to do something, anything to
help—whether out of a sense of what was morally just, or
out of religious or personal guilt, or fear of eventual retribution—as long as they did not have to reach out into
those needy communities themselves with their own
clean, well-manicured hands.

They were far preferable, at least, to their most visible
alternatives, the outright bigots who angrily bemoaned my
presence. To them, I was the reason their sons did not get
into Harvard. Perhaps they imagined I was another tenth
baby born out of wedlock who would someday have ten
illegitimate children myself and thus take over the world by
outbreeding white people. Or I was the beneficiary of
Head Start, food stamps, and other expensive government-
sponsored entitlement programs that siphoned off their tax
dollars. I was responsible for the resurgence of tuberculosis
in the United States, the illegal immigrant who smuggled
the organism into the country hidden in my lungs like con-
traband. I was not human to them, so I myself could not
suffer; I was simply a vector. I was all the potentially lethal
vermin and the terrible scourges they carried, the fierce
African killer bee, the ravenous Medfly, the repulsive cock-
roach, the blood-sucking mosquito, the typhus-infected
rat. I was the pathetic monkey trying to imitate them, to
steal their precious American know-how and cutting-edge
technology and take it back to my own country. I was drag-

ging their gloriously free society down the tubes, by taking insatiable advantage of and twisting that same freedom to serve my own selfish purposes. Sadly—and this seemed to be the extent of their emotional response to the remotely uncomfortable problem of my assumed to be impoverished existence—I could never be as smart, or as productive, or as innovative as they were. Only my inherent genetic deficiencies were to blame. Pseudo-Darwinian theories of survival and genetic advantagedness explained everything, and at the same time were conveniently thought to be unchangeable natural laws—while I knew that some of the audacious researchers among these most dangerous of my enemies paradoxically attempted to manipulate human genes to cure cancer. I worried that perhaps someday I myself might become an unwilling subject in one of their diabolical experiments, my dissected rat brain floating in a great glass vat of saline, an anti-Frankenstein of sorts by whose gruesome disembodiment they hoped to salvage my least-impaired working parts and so re-engineer me into something more useful before discarding the rest. In my overactive imagination, I envisioned them as high-powered "mad scientists" who secretly hoped that by their ultrasophisticated genetic techniques they could purge the human race of all its debilitating differences.

Then there were the few other Latinos in medicine whom I encountered, mostly older, disgruntled men who worked in chronically under funded, technology-poor primary care settings. Their own bitter intolerance for points of view discordant with their own sometimes shocked me.

I recall vividly the harrowing experience of an interview with the director of minority recruitment and retention at one West Coast medical school, who demanded to know why I had not checked any of the boxes next to the various categories that allowed the school to identify disadvantaged minority candidates. He implied that either I was ashamed of my heritage or I was a sellout too eager for the promised assimilation that would never come. When I tried to defend myself, on the basis that I was not sure I qualified for this special consideration, since I was ambivalent about whether I had been in any way truly disadvantaged—indeed, on some of my applications where the question was worded differently I *had* checked the box in question—he attacked me again, saying it was not special consideration but redress of past inequities that the admissions process was attempting to effect in its application review process. He then accused me of possibly the worst of all crimes, namely, the abandonment of my own "community." And so I was banished from the comforting embrace of my own people, before I had ever found the strength in their warm arms in the first place.

These three disparate but oddly complementary views of the community of origin to which I might belong only partially accounted for my resistance to the altruistic imperative of "giving back." That Latino cultures are stereotypically seen as welcoming, colorful, and musical made my perceived rejection by such a world when I finally came out as a gay man all the more painful and incomprehensible. The quietly closed doors and withheld invitations of the Anglo world paled in comparison with all those melodramatic and exaggerated tears, the near-violent disowning of my lover by his father, and the various sanctimonious sermons from Catholic priests that I endured when I was surrounded by Latinos, by my own family. Spanish words, because of their melodious gentleness, which allowed me to carry them closer to my heart, were much more capable of inflicting mortal wounds when turned against me. The Latino "community" fostered, to my surprise, a greater innate hostility to homosexuality, yet it was also the one place where I was supposed to be unconditionally loved. I reacted to its renunciation of me with a particularly potent mixture of anger and alienation. I began to think of myself as the most desperate of desperados: I was doubly illegal and doubly an ingrate, at once the unwanted and detestable immigrant who would disappoint the great nation that had reluctantly taken me in, and the repugnant and sinful castaway who would give us all a bad name, who would shame the very culture that had given me life. After all, we as a people were too poor for such an extravagance of love, an excessive love that was more like a sickness and so must have penetrated me during my adventures in the decadent white world.

Ironically, it was this unspeakable love that ultimately led me to the place where I am now, to a career not in diagnostic radiology but in general internal medicine, which allows me to provide primary care mostly to Latino patients in Boston. It was the love of another man, Latino himself, who taught me to love my culture, which led me to my place at the banquet table. It was his nurturing that sustained me through the cold winters of my New England college and later through the chilling anatomy labs of medical school. It did not matter to him whether on occasion I listened to old Broadway show tunes or to Led Zeppelin instead of salsa; we could still communicate in Spanish, we could still cook paella, or *plátanos* and rice and beans, and then discuss politics late into the night while chain-smoking cigarettes. I was forgiven for my awkward mispronunciations, in both English and Spanish, because bilingualism for us came to mean that my tongue was sometimes wrapped around his. We created our own country of origin, crossed oceans to our own undiscovered continent, wrote anthems for our own America the Fabulous. We planned to create a new life together in blissful harmony in Cuba someday—the choice of that most impossible and unimaginable of all locations was not exactly accidental—reclaiming my grandfather's lost plantation as our own, liberating it from the centuries of both capitalist and communist oppression. We would invent our own utopian political system, we would make idealistic lyrics like Martí's the law of the land. We who belonged neither to Spain nor to the United States, but to one another.

Under the tutelage of his love, I began to understand democracy and human rights in a revolutionary way. I saw particularly that in illness, as in desire, all people were indeed created equal. Suffering did not respect national boundaries or speak in only one approved language. The color of blood in every flag was monotonously the same unfathomable red. Need paid no attention to what part of

whose body was placed where. Death visited every neighborhood, riding in on the subway or in a stretch limousine
at any hour of the day or night. Though wealth might
have the power to promote health, and maybe even to
prolong life, in the end all my patients needed me to hold
their hands, or to smile and to touch their faces. Everyone
needed a witness; all of them wanted someone to whom
they could tell their final stories. Afterward, the agonal last
breaths always followed the same basic pattern, and the
flat green line on the monitor always failed to be rekindled
with the electrical waveform of a beating heart.

Oppression, too, became even more physically embodied, all the more obvious in the quotidian lives of my
patients, to whose suffering I was finally awakened. The
infected rat bite, the debilitating toxic exposure, and the
relentless spread of AIDS were no longer simply the documentation of losses that I had learned, from the history of
my own family, to compile passively, losses about which
nothing could be done; rather, each became a form of active
violence perpetrated by the powerful against the weak, calling for an immediate, drastic, and equally purposeful
response. I began to understand how one atrocity led to
another: from the genocide of this land's indigenous peoples
(a fact I had once haughtily questioned) where European
diseases were literally employed as weapons against native
people, to the murder and starvation of *mejicanos* and *cali-
fornios* who remained in their homes after Mexico ceded its
northern territories to the United States, to the ongoing
American embargo of Cuba, where because of the lack of
vaccines and antibiotics children continue to die each day.

I learned from reading the newspapers many things that were never mentioned in my medical textbooks. I witnessed that the health care policy of the moment was being shaped by the same aggressive impulses to control and to subjugate other people that had led to the wars and the destruction of the not-so-distant past. The contentious debates over funding to combat AIDS raged in ever more hostile terms during my four years of medical school. It was for all intents and purposes a war, one which had led desperate and misguided ACT UP members to interrupt a Catholic mass by blocking the aisles of Saint Patrick's Cathedral in New York and spitting out the host, and one where the rhetoric of hate and bigotry has had its most venomous expression from Jesse Helms, the senior Republican senator from North Carolina, who spoke the following words of enlightenment on the Senate floor:

> What originally began as a measured response to a public
> health emergency has become a weapon, frankly, for the
> deterioration of America's Judeo-Christian value system.
> There's not a chance this bill will be stopped because there's
> a powerful lobby out there in the media and in the homo-
> sexual community, and senators are scrambling to put their
> names on anything that has to do with AIDS.
>
> (The Associated Press, 1990)

Weapon, community, homosexual, America, values, Judeo-Christian, AIDS. Was my community after all "the homosexual community" that Jesse Helms seemed so adept at identifying and annihilating while I, one of its own members, had struggled so long to find it? Did my assent to this

question therefore mean that I was not American? Or not
Christian? Or not Latino? These questions about labels
began to swirl in my head as I made my rounds in the hospital each morning, and though their answers might seem
obvious, my education and my pride in my accomplish-
ments rose to a painful hard knot in my throat as I stared
into the eyes of those who were actually dying, those
gaunt men and women who were neither senators nor
physicians, those people who asked me quietly in Spanish
for a glass of water before I left, those who were not necessarily gay or Latino, or heterosexual or African American
or female or white; their most conspicuous defining char-
acteristic was that they were *suffering*. How convenient, I
thought, that the same terrible disease could be used to
decimate minority cultures and simultaneously to destroy
the values of the much stronger mainstream.

I have come to appreciate how little one's own sense of
identity ultimately seems to matter in the definition of
communities, in the drawing of national or sexual or linguistic boundaries, when such tremendously powerful
adversarial forces are at work. Out there somewhere in the
larger culture, whether in an institutionalized form of
human nature that insists on separating us into digestible
groups or as an aggregate of individual human choices to
know only one version of any story, there must exist a prin-
ciple by which all are probed and assigned a place. Because
my training is both in medicine and in poetry, because my
languages are both English and Spanish, because my love is
at once conventional and queer, and because I was born in
only one place and at one moment in time, I once had this

fantasy: the invention of a single blood test whose undeni-able result could be related and understood by anyone in a few spoken words and then sealed with a kiss, a test that proved beyond all doubt that we were all fundamentally the same creatures. I have seen our naked bodies, so often the instruments or the objects of our divisions; I know I am just as human as Tom Cruise, whose beautiful image is worth millions of dollars, just as human as my IV drug-using AIDS patient in the ER whose name I forgot proba-bly within minutes of her death in my arms. I freely admit I am still naive, believing at times that a touch can heal even in an ICU, or that a prayer can be heard well outside the confines of a church.

It has been suggested to me that my biggest problem, however it is defined, has resulted from an exaggerated capacity on my part for sensing the innumerable wrongs done to me. I have been told that I must always remember how to forget. The organs of my voice have become hypertrophied from saying the same things over and over again to a world that refuses to listen; no matter how hard I try, I will never re-create the Aztec canon or the Mayan system of arithmetic. And enough with the queer thing, they say, warning me that I am beginning to sound like the frustrated mariachi who wants to wear his pink ruffled shirt to sing in a restaurant that serves only tacos. Too serious, too sensitive, too insistent, my parents say. My poems have an unfortunate tendency to wallow in the misery of their own creation, besides being obsessed with my patri-archal past. Perhaps I have driven the members of my com-munity, whoever they might be, away from me with my

unending questions and saturnine social skills. Perhaps I
have told one too many a story about a patient whose life
or death changed my own. If these criticisms are accurate,
then I accept them; but since even before my awkward
conversation with the dean, really since the moment I realized I shared the world with other people, sometimes in
spite of myself and sometimes with the fullest of hearts, I
have felt compelled to search for some way to give.

Once I felt that the most insurmountable of all the
obstacles facing me in the care of my patients was my own
selfishness. I was too busy to listen to the pathetic story of
another person's suffering, too hungry to stay a few minutes later to comfort another person in need, too important to be burdened with another person's trivial concern.
The next great hurdle I encountered also had to do with
the imperilment of empathy: will the heart of my seventy-
five-year-old grandmother of eight from Guatemala with
congestive heart failure finally burst when she learns that I
am gay? (She cried the same tears as my own grandmother once did, and revealed to me that one of her own grandchildren was a lesbian.) I have tried to internalize what I
have learned from my patients themselves. I remember
how they have endured, and how they have taught me
what I once thought was impossible, something I thought
I might never learn: the limitless ways that I can give back
to many communities.

I wonder whom you would see if I were to come to you
for help. What would you give me? I am not tall, I have an
olive complexion, I have dark straight hair, I have green
eyes. I am a bit overweight, I have a job, I have enough

money for shelter, for food. I look like the hybrid that I am. Like most hybrids, I will never reproduce. I am toxic to my own aspirations and dreams; in my veins run both the promise of a better life and its incessant denial. My physical appearance marks me now, though it remains unmarred, unlike the bodies of so many others of my kind. I walk down the street in San Francisco, and I am mistaken for a Mexican. I could be illegal. Once an elderly, blue-veined, American lady driving a white Cadillac asked me whether I was Jewish. I thought she recognized me. I am the Jew of the Caribbean—isn't that what they call Cubans? My mother was born in Dover, New Jersey. Her parents' relatives still live in Italy, that's what they always said. My father is a U.S. citizen, but I never asked him where he keeps his documentation. I should know that. We memorized an American version of his own history. Maybe I can give that back. Maybe I can teach you to love something new, like salsa or black beans and white rice or Gloria Estefan or Andy García or Celia Cruz or Albita. I want you to know something about me, about us, after you finish reading this. I am writing a new poem later today. I want you to read it, too. I want to be mistaken for your brother, or your son; I want to remind you of your daughter, your mother, your sister. I want to give you something, not a disease, but perhaps a cure. I want you to look into the liquid mirror of my eyes, and see someone you recognize. Someone you have always known, someone you might even love.

Yourself.